Optimum
Nutrition
for Your
Child's Mind

Optimum Nutrition

for Your Child's Mind

Maximize Your Child's Potential

Patrick Holford
and Deborah Colson

CELESTIAL ARTS
Berkeley | Toronto

All supplements should be kept out of reach of infants and young children.

Celestial Arts
an imprint of Ten Speed Press
PO Box 7123
Berkeley, California 94707
www.tenspeed.com

Distributed in Canada by Ten Speed Press Canada.

First published in the United Kingdom in 2005 by Piatkus, an imprint of Little, Brown Book Group Ltd.

Cover and text design by Chloe Rawlins

Library of Congress Cataloging-in-Publication Data
Holford, Patrick.
  Optimum nutrition for your child's mind : maximize your child's potential / Patrick Holford and Deborah Colson.
      p. cm.
  Includes bibliographical references and index.
  Summary: "A science-based guide to understanding how choosing the right foods (and avoiding the wrong ones) can boost your child's intelligence and improve mood and behavior"—Provided by publisher.
  ISBN 978-1-58761-332-6
  1. Children—Nutrition. 2. Intellect—Nutritional aspects. 3. Pediatric neuropsychology. 4. Nootropic agents. I. Colson, Deborah. II. Title.
  RJ206.H745 2008
  618.92—dc22
                                 2008007067

Printed in the United States of America
First printing, 2008

1 2 3 4 5 6 7 8 9 10 — 12 11 10 09 08

Contents

PART 1—FOOD FOR THE BRAIN

PART 2—GIVE YOUR CHILD A HEAD START

PART 3—SOLVING PROBLEMS

PART 4—FOOD FOR THOUGHT

Acknowledgments

W e'd like to thank the many scientists whose studies we have quoted, who have tirelessly put the role of optimum nutrition for children's brain development on the map, often funding their own research. Enormous thanks go to Susannah Lawson, coauthor of *Optimum Nutrition Before, During and After Pregnancy*, for her many contributions. But, most of all, we'd like to thank the many children and their parents whom we've worked with at the Brain Bio Centre: it is they who have taught us the most.

GUIDE TO ABBREVIATIONS, MEASURES, AND REFERENCES

ABBREVIATIONS AND MEASURES

> 1 gram (g) = 1,000 milligrams (mg) =
> 1,000,000 micrograms (mcg, also written μg)

All vitamins are measured in milligrams or micrograms. Vitamins A, D, and E can also be measured in International Units (IUs), a measurement designed to standardize the various forms of these vitamins that have different potencies.

100 IU of vitamin A = 30.3 mcg	100 IU of vitamin D = 2.5 mcg
100 IU of vitamin E = 67 mg	
1 pound (lb) = 16 ounces (oz)	2.2 lb = 1 kilogram (kg)
1 pint = 0.47 liters	2.11 pints = 1 liter

In this book calories means kilocalories (kcals).

REFERENCES AND FURTHER SOURCES OF INFORMATION

Hundreds of references from respected scientific literature have been used in the writing of this book. Details of specific studies referred to are listed on pages 220–238. On page 213 you will find a list of the best books to read to enable you to dig more deeply into the topics covered. The Resources section on pages 214–219 provides details on support organizations, suppliers of good-quality supplements and laboratory tests, as well as details of organizations that can help you find a nutritionist in your area. In this book, a nutritionist is defined as a professional who would give the advice in this book and be able to recommend supplements. A nutritionist could be an ND (naturopathic doctor), MD (medical doctor), or RN (nurse practitioner). Your nutritionist should be able to run blood tests or refer you to a doctor who can.

Introduction

All parents have an instinct to help their children be all they can. We want our children to be happy, intelligent, and resourceful, with the full range of life skills they'll need to live productively and well. That is, in essence, what childhood is all about.

We teach our children how to eat, how to walk and talk, how to get the most out of what they're learning in school. We give them as much love and attention as we can to enable them to develop physically, mentally, and emotionally. We read books about parenting, we try not to make the same mistakes our parents made, we struggle over choosing the right school to support our children through the process of becoming adults and finding their way in the world.

But through all of this, do we really take into account the fact that every step children take—whether it's their first toddle on the kitchen floor or their sudden plunge into emotions and relationships as teenagers— depends on how well their brains are working? And that that, in turn, depends in large part on how well their brain is nourished?

FROM PLATE TO BRAIN

This is a how-to book. Whether your child is one year old or fifteen, you want to know what you can do to help her be all she can be—and you'll discover how in these pages. Armed with more than twenty years' experience of working with children, we are going to show you, step-by-step, what optimum nutrition for your child's mind really means.

At long last, governments and schools are realizing children's need for a truly well-balanced diet rather than the junk food afterthought they've had to put up with. Society is waking up to the fact that schools have a moral responsibility to give children good food and that the quality of school meals has long been too low a priority.

Why has this grim state of affairs persisted so long? Simply because food has been misperceived as fuel so that, if a child is full after a meal and isn't showing obvious signs of malnourishment, it's seen as "good enough."

But the true picture lies in how you read the signs in a child's behavior or appearance. Take intelligence. Somehow embedded in our culture is the false idea that this is inherited and there's nothing you can do about it. I (Patrick) trained as a psychologist, and I've always had a keen interest in our intellectual development. As the brain is essentially manufactured from the food we eat, I was already wondering back in the 1980s whether giving children extra vitamins and minerals could boost their intelligence.

Working with secondary school head Gwillym Roberts and Professor David Benton from the University of Wales in Swansea, we proved that you can dramatically boost children's IQs just by making changes in their nutrition—an experiment showcased in a 1988 BBC documentary. In the study, we measured the IQ scores of ninety schoolchildren and then gave thirty of them a high-dose multivitamin, thirty a dummy pill, and thirty nothing. After eight months, we reevaluated their IQs. Only those children on the vitamins had a staggering increase in their IQs of over 10 points![1]

This study, the first of its kind anywhere in the world, raised a new question: how can you keep your child's mind optimally nourished?

NUTRITION IN MIND

If there is a difference between the learning and behavior of kids who eat junk food with abandon and those who are following the so-called well-balanced diet, what is that difference, why is there a difference, and what exactly should you, as a parent, be feeding your child? These are the questions we've lived and breathed for the past twenty years.

As you'll see in this book, study after study shows that you can increase intelligence, attention span, concentration, problem-solving ability, emotional response, mood, physical coordination—all the facets of intelligence—simply by changing what goes into and onto their bowls, plates, and lunch boxes.

While the practical advice we'll be giving you is based on solid scientific research, we feel even more confident about our conclusions because we have worked with hundreds of children over the past two decades.

Some of them were disabled, some coping with serious behavioral problems, yet all were transformed once their own unique optimum nutrition needs were discovered and fulfilled.

Every day at the London clinic of the Brain Bio Centre, part of the Food for the Brain charity founded by Patrick, we see children who are struggling to learn, develop, and adapt. I (Deborah) am a clinical nutritionist specializing in children's development. My job is not only to find out what's wrong—be it a food allergy, a chemical sensitivity, or a nutrient deficiency—but also to show parents how to make good food that children like, weaning them off sugar and expanding the range of healthful foods on the daily menu.

As well as working one to one with kids and parents at the Brain Bio Centre, we've tested our theories in primary schools, secondary schools, and special schools for disadvantaged children. A leading British morning television program, for example, gave us one week to improve the learning of a class of seven- to eight-year-olds. Later on you'll read the story of Reece, a "hyperactive" child in this class whose reading level went up a year in one month on the diet.

Tonight with Trevor McDonald, an investigative news program, gave us three badly behaved boys, all of whom had been kicked out of mainstream schools, and asked us to get them back on track in a month. You'll find out what happened to one of these boys (see case study, page 124), along with the supplements we've recommended for all these kids, and how a simple test can reveal whether your child's brain is working at its best (see "B Deficiencies—the Homocysteine Link," pages 61–62).

In 2005, we founded a UK-based charity to promote the link between nutrition and mental health. The charity, Food for the Brain, conducted a survey of over 10,000 children in Britain comparing food intake with academic performance, behavior, and health. The children were of all ages, with three-quarters of them aged from six to fifteen years old. The survey, the largest ever in Britain, found that more than one in three children in the survey had problems behaving and performing academically, and there was a strong association between poor eating habits and poor behavior and academic performance. A number of key foods were identified as having a substantially beneficial effect on both behavior and academic performance.

Some key findings of the survey were:

- Children who eat diets high in fried food or take-out food are three times more likely to be badly behaved.
- Children who eat vegetables, oily fish, nuts, and seeds do best in school.
- Children on the best diets have 11 percent higher scores in national exams than those on the worst diets.
- The best foods for behavior are fruit and vegetables—those children eating the most of both are twice as likely to be well behaved.

The worst foods are fried, take-out, and processed food, microwave meals, and sugar.

- An amazing 44 percent of children who eat this type of junk food most days suffer from bad behavior, compared with only 16 percent of children who never eat fried or take-out food.
- Children who ate nuts and seeds daily did twice as well academically as children who didn't eat nuts and seeds at all.
- The best foods for good national exam scores are dark green leafy vegetables, oily fish, and water. The worst foods are processed foods and microwave meals.

We would expect these findings to be similar across the Western world.

Much of our work has been with children and young adults diagnosed with ADHD, autism, Asperger's, depression, and even psychosis. The usual route for children with these conditions is prescription drugs or specialized psychological support. We believe that optimum nutrition is a vital aspect of helping these children discover, or recover, their full potential. Consider these studies:

- A research team at the University of Michigan found that iron deficiency in infancy was associated with worse performances in intelligence tests up to nineteen years later.[2]
- Bernard Gesch, director of the UK charity Natural Justice, gave some of Britain's worst juvenile offenders supplements of vitamins,

minerals, and essential fats, or placebos, and demonstrated a dramatic 35 percent decrease in aggressive acts only in those taking the supplements.[3]

- Dr. Alexandra Richardson of the University of Oxford, UK, conducted a randomized controlled trial with 117 children aged five to twelve years who had coordination problems. The children who received supplements of omega-3 and omega-6 fatty acids showed significant improvements in reading, spelling, and behavior over three months compared to those who didn't receive the supplements.[4]
- Researchers from Örebro University in Sweden compared the school grades in ten core subjects with homocysteine levels in a group of 692 school children aged nine to fifteen. (Homocysteine is an indicator of B vitamin deficiency.) Higher homocysteine levels were strongly associated with lower grades.[5]
- Researchers at the Institute of Child Health in London placed seventy-eight hyperactive children on a "few foods" diet, which eliminates both chemical additives and common food allergens. The behavior of fifty-nine of the children, or 76 percent, improved during this open trial. To check whether the foods would affect the children's behavior if no one knew whether they were eating them or not, the researchers managed to disguise the foods and additives that provoked reactions in nineteen of the children. When these children were given the disguised offending foods, their behavior ratings and performance in psychological testing both worsened.[6]

If simple changes in nutrition can have such profound effects on the young people in these studies, isn't it likely that optimum nutrition can help your child reach her full potential? That means every child—not just children with conditions such as autism, hyperactivity, or behavioral problems. Optimum nutrition can sharpen up your child's mind and mood even if you feel she is doing "all right."

As you follow the guidelines in this book, you will notice gradual improvements in your child's ability to learn and behave. You really can change how your child thinks, feels, and behaves by changing what goes into her mouth, and we're going to show you how.

By doing so, you'll be in the vanguard of teachers, health professionals, and other concerned parents who are leading a revolution in food awareness. Although governments are waking up to the implications of all the new research, they have not yet accepted across the board just how profoundly nutrition can influence learning and behavior.

The time is ripe for change, and you can help make it happen.

HOW TO USE THIS BOOK

In part 1, **Food for the Brain**, you'll discover the five essential brain foods, an optimum intake of which is essential for maximizing your child's potential. There are also five "antinutrients" that can disrupt and damage the brain and are best avoided. This part shows you what to feed your child, and what to avoid.

In part 2, **Give Your Child a Head Start**, you'll discover the foods and supplements that are proven to boost IQ, improve mood and behavior, sharpen memory and concentration, and improve reading and writing. In this part of the book, you will discover how to maximize your child's potential for better school performance, happiness, and personal fulfillment.

In part 3, **Solving Problems**, we give you nutritional solutions for children with conditions such as autism, hyperactivity, and aggression to help you maximize their potential for mental and emotional health.

In part 4, **Food for Thought**, we'll show you how to put this into action, explaining what to do to feed your child properly, from infancy to teenage years. You'll find plenty of shopping tips, meal ideas, and practical ways of keeping your child's diet on track, as well as advice on how to choose the right supplements.

The biggest gift we can give our children is getting them off to the best start in life, socially and academically. A huge part of that is to make available to them the best nutrition, to help them feel alert, energetic, happy, and unstressed, with a clear mind and a focused intelligence. This book is written with that goal in mind.

Wishing you and your children the best of health,

—Patrick Holford and Deborah Colson

PART 1

Food for the Brain

Food directly affects how your child thinks and feels because his brain (and yours) is made of it. There are five essential brain foods: slow-release carbohydrates, essential fats, phospholipids, amino acids, and vitamins and minerals. An optimum intake of these is essential for maximizing your child's potential. Then there are the five "antinutrients," substances that can disrupt and damage the brain—refined sugar, damaged fats, certain chemical food additives, toxic minerals, and food allergens. These are best avoided. In this part of the book, you'll find out what, and what not, to feed your child.

Chapter 1

How Food Builds the Brain

One of the most limiting concepts in the human sciences is the idea that mind and body are separate. Try asking an anatomist, a psychologist, and a biochemist where the mind begins and the body ends. It is a stupid question, and yet that is exactly what modern science has done by separating psychology from medicine. Few psychologists know much about brain chemistry and the importance of nutrition, and few doctors know enough about the psychological or nutritional factors that affect a child's development.

But it's not just the scientists who live by this false dichotomy. It's all of us. It's undoubtedly second nature to you to help your child grow physically strong and healthy. But when he's concentrating poorly, behaving badly, or struggling to read, does poor nourishment cross your mind? If it doesn't, it's vital to know that all these attributes and behaviors are governed by a network of interconnecting brain cells, each of which depends profoundly on what your child puts into his mouth.

Many of our children are struggling to keep up. They're living with constant tiredness, inattention, erratic behavior, anxiety, stress, depression, and sleeping problems. Too many children are suffering from mental health problems ranging from attention deficit disorder to autism, hyperactivity, and dyslexia; or they're simply not achieving their full potential in school and at home because the way they feel makes it difficult to focus and learn. In fact, the world over there's been a massive rise in the incidence of mental health problems, especially among young people.[1]

By understanding how your child's brain works, you can eradicate these problems and smooth your child's path through his crucial developing years. It will become more than clear why giving a child certain nutrients every day, ideally from birth, can have a profound effect on how he thinks and feels, and thus how he behaves in the here and now and how he develops over time.

BRAINS—WHAT MAKE US HUMAN

Our story starts not at birth but at conception and all the way through pregnancy. Studies of the time we spend in the womb are showing us that human growth and development—unlike that of, say, a rhinoceros—center largely on the development of the brain. Brains, not brawn, are what make us human.

For example, a human baby's brain is more than 300 times larger, compared to its body size, than that of a rhinoceros. Size is important, but that's not all. During development in the womb, half of all the nutrition the fetus receives from its mother is directly channeled into feeding brain growth.

This is quite a task. Although a mere 1 pound in weight at birth, your child's brain consumes, and needs, a vast quantity of nutrients, including proteins, carbohydrates, vitamins, minerals, and essential fats. Fats are a big one here, as the brain is literally made out of it. In fact, if you drained all the water out of a brain, a whopping 60 percent of it would be fat.

Four specific kinds of fat, known as AA, DHA, EPA, and DGLA (more on these later), make up 20 percent of the brain. So deficiencies of these at any time, but especially during fetal or early development, can have profound repercussions on intelligence and behavior.

So vital are these fats to the growing fetus that it will literally rob its mother's brain to make its own. It's a case of "Mommy, I shrunk your brain": if a pregnant woman's diet is deficient in the essential fats, her brain will actually get smaller!

At every stage of brain development, achieving optimum nutrition is essential to guarantee that your child achieves his full potential. At birth, the level of essential fats in the umbilical cord of a newborn infant correlates with the speed of his thinking at age eight. By the age of eight, the blood level of homocysteine, which is the best indicator of a child's B vitamin status, will correlate with his school grades.[2] If a teenager's daily intake of zinc is just twice the level of the recommended daily allowance (RDA), this can improve attention and concentration to an astonishing degree.[3] And at any age, the intake of antinutrients like sugar and damaged fats has proven harmful effects on both learning and behavior.

If you find these facts hard to believe, you may not be aware how flexible and open to change the human brain is. Let's look at it for a moment to understand why this is.

JOINED-UP THINKING

As it grows, a fetus builds thousands of brain cells, called neurons, every minute. By the age of two, a child's brain has approximately 100 billion of them. That's a lot—approximately the same number of neurons as there are trees in the Amazon! And just like the interlocking branches of those billions of rain forest trees, the neurons are connected up. So what we call the brain is essentially a network of these specialized nerve cells, all linked up to other neurons.

While the number of neurons doesn't increase in children beyond the age of two, the number of connections made between neurons does, very dramatically. When a baby is born, every neuron in the cerebral cortex—the gray matter and outermost layer of the brain—can connect with about 2,500 other neurons. By the time that child is two or three years old, that number has swollen to 15,000.

These connections are vital to memory, cognition, and learning because they're the conduits along which the electrical impulses of our thoughts travel. And children, those master learners, are hard wiring these connections every minute.

When learning language, for instance, young children will keep repeating words to hard wire the image they are seeing with the sound they are making, reinforced by your positive feedback. Every thought they think is represented by a ripple of activity across the network of neurons. With repeated thoughts and actions, be it speech or movement, the neuronal pathways are reinforced. Meanwhile, other, redundant connections will get dismantled. Unlike other organs in the body, the brain is always restructuring itself.

Let's take a closer look at the connections between neurons. Neurons have branches called dendrites, and where one dendrite meets another, there's a gap, like the spark gap in a spark plug. This gap is called a synapse, and it's across it that messages are sent from one neuron to another.

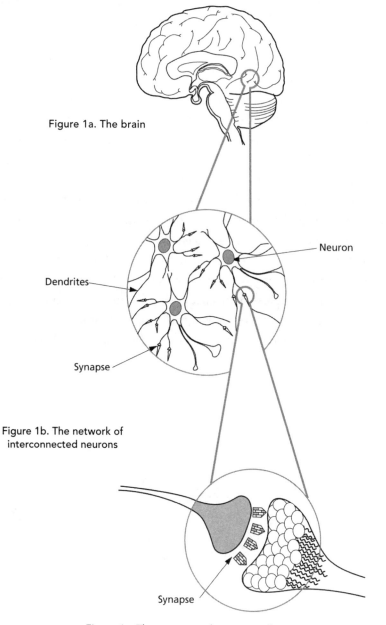

Figure 1a. The brain

Neuron

Dendrites

Synapse

Figure 1b. The network of interconnected neurons

Synapse

Figure 1c. The synapse, where two cells meet

The message is sent from a sending station and received in a receiving station, called a receptor. These sending and receiving stations are built out of essential fats, found in fish and seeds; phospholipids, present in eggs and organ meats; and amino acids, the raw material of protein.

The message itself, known as a neurotransmitter, is in most cases made out of amino acids. Different amino acids make different neurotransmitters. For example, the neurotransmitter serotonin, which keeps you happy, is made from the amino acid tryptophan. Adrenaline and dopamine, which keep you motivated, are made from phenylalanine.

Turning an amino acid into a neurotransmitter is no simple job. Enzymes in the brain that depend on vitamins, minerals, and special amino acids accomplish this task. These vitamins and minerals also control the steady supply of fuel—blood sugar or glucose—that powers each neuron.

From all this, you can see how the food your child eats does more than build his body. It's building the very structure of his brain, from the neurons themselves to the messages that shoot from one to another. So food governs how your child thinks and feels to a critical degree.

The basic structure of your child's brain is laid down by genetics. But what you feed him, along with what he learns, helps develop that structure, and through that his intelligence and ability to learn, adapt, and have a happy and fulfilling life. While you can't change genes, you can change your child's nutrition and learning resources. That's why your biggest task,

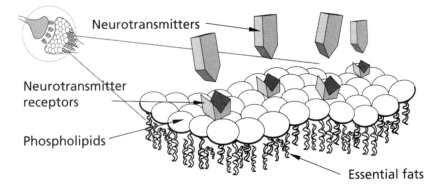

Figure 2. Close-up of a receptor

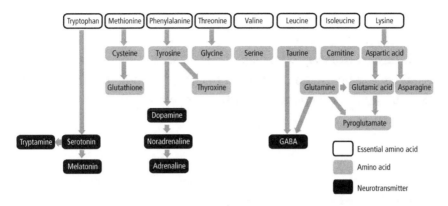

Figure 3. Neurotransmitters, made from amino acids

as a parent, is ensuring optimum nutrition while stimulating your child's built-in capacity for learning.

In the context of your child's brain, optimum nutrition is all about choosing five essential foods and avoiding others. Let's look at them now.

WHAT GOES ON—OR OFF—THE PLATE

Optimum nutrition means achieving the right intake of the five essential brain foods:

- Balanced blood sugar—the brain's superfuel
- Essential fats—why a "fathead" is a smart head
- Phospholipids—memory molecules that give oomph to the brain
- Amino acids—the brain's messengers
- Vitamins and minerals—the intelligent nutrients that keep the brain in tune

But this isn't the whole story. You will also need to avoid antinutrients—substances that damage the brain:

- Refined sugar—carbohydrates robbed of essential nutrients
- Damaged fats—from fried food to hydrogenated fats
- Toxic minerals—from copper to mercury
- Chemical food additives—colorings, flavorings, and preservatives
- Food allergens—common foods your child might be allergic to

In the chapters that follow we'll explain how to discover which foods or chemicals your child is particularly sensitive to and would do best to avoid. And the next five chapters explain in detail what the five essential brain foods are and how to give your child the optimal amount. These chapters explain the basics of optimum nutrition for your child's mind.

Chapter 2

No Sugar, Thanks— I'm Sweet Enough Already

Have you ever picked your child up from a birthday party and opened the door to a roomful of kids bouncing off the walls? All that sugar has an amazingly dramatic effect on the brain. So it's hardly surprising that in daily life, too, overdoing the sweet stuff affects your child's behavior.

Yet nothing is more important for your child's brain than sugar—blood sugar, or glucose, that is. It's the brain's main fuel, so without an adequate supply we can't think clearly. We get it from the sugars and starches—in other words, the carbohydrates—in the foods we eat. The trick lies in keeping that supply even.

Too much sugar, and you get the wall-bouncing effect. Too little, and your child could experience symptoms like fatigue, irritability, dizziness, insomnia, aggression, anxiety, sweating (especially at night), poor concentration, excessive thirst, depression, crying spells, or blurred vision. So for your child to be able to think with clarity and behave rationally, it's vital that her glucose supply stays steady and even.

John is a case in point. Four-year-old John's parents brought him to see us at the Brain Bio Centre because they were concerned about his severe speech and language delay and his inability to concentrate. We screened him for various biochemical imbalances and analyzed his diet. John's diet, while fairly typical for a four-year-old and not especially unhealthy, contained a lot of hidden sugar, so we recommended that his parents reduce all sources of sugar as much as possible, including high-sugar fruits such as bananas. Within a few weeks, John was a different child according to his parents, babysitter, and teachers. His scribbling had transformed into drawings accompanied by a verbal explanation. He slept better at night and no longer needed to nap during the day, was much calmer, had improved comprehension, and began attempting jigsaw puzzles. As if to illustrate how sensitive John is to sugar, one day during this period, John's granddad gave him half a banana, thinking it was allowed on the diet and the effect was incredible. "He went completely nuts," his mother told us, and literally ran from one end of the house to the other for an hour until the effect of the banana wore off. No chance of any sneaky sugar from doting grandparents again!

Check your child out on the questionnaire below.

Blood Sugar Check

Does your child:

- ❑ Usually eat white bread, rice, or pasta instead of brown or whole-grain?
- ❑ Crave sugar, candy, or refined carbohydrates such as chocolate, cookies, toast and jelly, or sweetened cereals?
- ❑ Have sugary foods or drinks at regular intervals during the day?
- ❑ Crave caffeinated drinks such as sodas?
- ❑ Sometimes skip meals, especially breakfast?
- ❑ Seem to be slow to get going in the morning?
- ❑ Have energy slumps during the day?
- ❑ Sometimes lose concentration or have poor attention span?
- ❑ Get dizzy, dopey, or irritable if she doesn't eat often?
- ❑ Seem to lack energy?

Check the box for each "yes" answer. If you check five or more, the chances are your child's blood sugar balance is less than perfect.

Later in this chapter, we're going to explain exactly what you need to do to improve your child's blood sugar balance and banish these symptoms. Bur first it helps to understand how blood sugar actually works. How does glucose get into the bloodstream, and how do you ensure the right amount ends up there and reaches your child's brain?

THE UPS AND DOWNS OF BLOOD SUGAR

As we saw above, the raw material of blood sugar is the carbohydrates in what you eat and drink. When your child eats carbohydrate-rich foods such as cereal, bread, pasta, potatoes, or rice, the sugars and starches in these foods are broken down into glucose during digestion. The glucose is then absorbed into the bloodstream. Some carbohydrates, particularly the refined kind found in white bread, are broken down and absorbed more quickly than others—more on this in a moment.

Refined sugar, often in the form of sucrose, is the type found in sugary drinks and cereals. Their breakdown and absorption into the bloodstream is even faster, because sucrose and glucose are almost the same thing.

When your child consumes a lot of fast-releasing carbohydrate all at once (say, in a soda and cookie, or white toast and jelly), her blood glucose levels will soar. Glucose is powerful stuff and can actually damage nerves and blood vessels. The body copes with this by enlisting the help of the hormone insulin, which is released from the pancreas when a burst of glucose hits the bloodstream.

Once in the blood, insulin escorts the glucose into cells, where it's used for energy. Any excess—and there will be if your child has overdosed on refined carbohydrates—is stored as glycogen in other parts of the body such as the muscles and liver. When these stores are full, any remaining glucose is converted to body fat.

In the sugar overdose scenario—after a big bowl of processed, sweetened cereal, or a box of candy at the movies, for example—the body responds to what it sees as a dangerous situation by releasing more insulin than normal. As a result, too much glucose can actually be escorted out of the bloodstream, leaving your child with too low a blood glucose level and a subsequent crash in energy. We've seen how nasty the symptoms of low blood glucose can be. But even worse, your child is then likely to crave more of what caused the problem in the first place—sugar—just to get rid of the unpleasant feelings. And round we go again. It's a vicious cycle that leads to more cravings, more extreme mood fluctuations, and progressively poorer concentration and behavior.

Sugar Imbalance and Your Child

Seesawing blood sugar levels not only affect your child's mood and behavior, they can also affect her IQ. Research at the Massachusetts Institute of Technology found a 25 percent difference between the IQ scores of children who were in the top fifth of the population for consumption of sugar and other refined carbohydrates and children who were in the bottom fifth.[1] So staying away from white bread, processed cereals, and sugar seems to be crucial to having a higher IQ.

But that's not all. To maximize mental performance, your child needs to have that all-important even supply of glucose to the brain; this has been well proven by Professor David Benton at Swansea University in the UK, who has found that dips in blood glucose are directly associated with poor attention, poor memory, and aggressive behavior.[2] Sugar has been implicated in aggressive behavior, anxiety, hyperactivity and attention deficit, depression, eating disorders, fatigue, and learning difficulties.[3]

Moreover, dietary studies consistently reveal that hyperactive children eat more sugar than other children and that reducing dietary sugar can halve disciplinary actions in juvenile delinquents.[4] A study of 265 hyperactive children found that more than three-quarters displayed abnormal glucose balance.[5]

INSIDE CARBOHYDRATES

We all need carbohydrates, and they're very important for your child. But as the evidence shows, you need to choose carefully which types she eats. Foods with complex carbohydrates, such as whole grains, vegetables, beans, or lentils, or with simpler carbohydrates such as fruit, take longer to digest than refined carbohydrates. As a result, the glucose released from these foods doesn't flood into the bloodstream but trickles in slowly over time; this means that it's used for energy rather than stored, leaving blood glucose levels on an even keel and preventing dramatic changes in mood, behavior, and energy.

Why Refined Is Bad

There's another reason why whole foods, such as whole oats, are better for you than foods rich in refined carbohydrates, such as white bread or pasta. By overprocessing carbohydrate foods, we are cheating nature, isolating the sweetness in the food and discarding the rest.

The most extreme example is concentrated sugar—white sugar, brown sugar, malt, glucose, honey, and corn syrup. These are fast-releasing, triggering a rapid rise in blood glucose levels, and at the same time almost completely devoid of vitamins and minerals. White sugar, for instance, is up to 90 percent lower in the vitamins and minerals present in the raw materials (such as beets) from which it was made. (More on the importance of vitamins and minerals in chapter 6.)

What about Fruit Sugar?

The main sugar in most fruit is the simple sugar fructose. Fructose enters the bloodstream fast but is classified as slow-releasing because the body has to convert it to glucose before it can be used as fuel, and this process slows down its effect on the body.

Some fruits, such as grapes and dates, contain almost pure glucose, putting the carbs they contain in the fast-releasing class. Apples, on the other hand, contain mainly fructose and so are classed as slow-releasing. Bananas contain both and raise blood glucose levels quite speedily. But all fresh fruit does have two big advantages. One is fiber, which slows down the release of the sugars contained in the fruit. The other is vitamins, which, as we'll see in chapter 6, are essential for physical and mental health.

What about dried fruit? It's problematic because it obviously has much less water than the same weight of fresh fruit, and this both concentrates the sugar and makes it much smaller and less filling—so you can end up

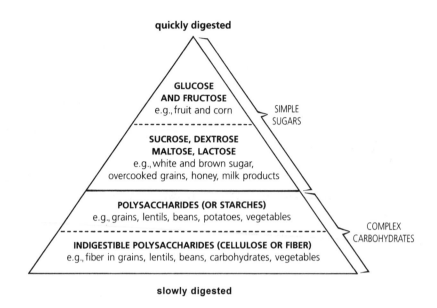

Figure 4. The sugar family

packing away quite a lot without realizing it. Moreover, the fiber in dried apples, for instance, is less effective in slowing down sugar release. So don't make dried fruit a substitute for fresh. And when you do give your child dried fruit, soak it first—when it's plumped up and rehydrated it will be more filling, so she's likely to eat less of it.

The Carbs That Keep Blood Sugar Even

Now that we know how important the release rate of carbohydrates is, how can you tell which are fast releasing and which are slow? As a general rule, you can assume that whole, unprocessed foods are the slowest to release their sugar. Beyond this, you can use a measure called glycemic load (GL). In essence, GL measures the effect of a food on blood glucose levels. GL takes into account both a food's glycemic index (a measure of whether its carbohydrates are fast- or slow-releasing, also known as GI) and how much carbohydrate it contains. Foods with a GL of less than 10 are good and should be the staple foods of your child's diet. A GL of 11 to 14 is okay and can be eaten in moderation. A GL higher than 15 should be avoided. Beware of combining two moderate-GL foods in one meal. When they're eaten together, their GL adds up to high. For example, whole-grain toast with unsweetened peanut butter (moderate with low GL) remains moderate, whereas a whole wheat pancake with maple syrup (moderate with high GL) shoots up.

The chart below gives the GL score of an average serving of a range of common foods. You can start to use this now by checking out what your child eats for breakfast. If she starts the day with puffed rice cereal and raisins, both of which have a high GL score, she's getting rocket fuel first thing in the morning, and that means that a couple of hours later her blood glucose, and energy, will plummet. But give her oatmeal sweetened with a chopped apple—both of which are slow releasing—and her energy and concentration will last right through to lunch.

Glycemic Load of Common Foods

Item	Serving size (in oz)	GL per serving
Baked Goods		
Bread, bagel, white	2.5	25
Bread, baguette, white, plain	1.1	15
Bread, flatbread, Middle Eastern	1.1	15
Bread, flatbread, wheat	1.1	10
Bread, gluten-free, fiber-enriched	1.1	9
Bread, gluten-free, multigrain	1.1	10
Bread, gluten-free, white	1.1	11
Bread, light rye	1.1	10
Bread, pita, white	1.1	10
Bread, pumpernickel	1.1	6
Bread, rice, high-amylose	1.1	7
Bread, rice, low-amylose	1.1	8
Bread, sourdough rye	1.1	6
Bread, white	1.1	10
Bread, white, high-fiber	1.1	9
Bread, whole-grain rye	1.1	8
Bread, whole wheat	1.1	9
Cake, banana, made without sugar	2.8	16
Cake, sponge, plain	2.2	17

(continued)

Glycemic Load of Common Foods, continued

Item	Serving size (in oz)	GL per serving
Cracker, rye crispbread	0.9	11
Cracker, water	0.9	13
Croissant	2.0	17
Doughnut, cake	1.6	17
Muffin, apple, made with sugar	2.1	13
Muffin, apple, made without sugar	2.1	9
Muffin, apple, oat, raisin, made from packaged mix	1.8	14
Muffin, blueberry	2.0	17
Muffin, bran	2.0	15
Muffin, carrot	2.0	20
Rice cakes, puffed	0.9	17
Tortilla, corn	1.8	12
Tortilla, wheat	1.8	8

Dairy Products

Item	Serving size (in oz)	GL per serving
Custard, homemade from milk	3.5	7
Ice cream, regular	1.8	8
Milk, condensed, sweetened	1.8	17
Milk, rice	8.8	14
Milk, skim	8.8	4
Milk, soy	8.8	7
Milk, soy (sweetened with apple juice concentrate)	8.8	8
Milk, soy (sweetened with sugar)	8.8	9
Milk, soy, 1.5 percent fat	8.8	8
Milk, whole	8.8	3
Yogurt, low-fat, fruit (with sugar)	7.0	10
Yogurt, nonfat (plain, no sugar)	7.0	3
Yogurt, plain (no sugar)	7.0	3
Yogurt, soy	7.0	7

Fruit

Item	Serving size (in oz)	GL per serving
Apples	4.2	6
Apples, dried	2.1	10
Apricots	4.2	5

Item	Serving size (in oz)	GL per serving
Apricots, canned in light syrup	4.2	12
Apricots, dried	2.1	9
Banana, raw	4.2	12
Blackberries	4.2	1
Blueberries	4.2	1
Cherries	4.2	3
Dates, dried	2.1	42
Figs, dried	2.1	16
Fruit cocktail, canned (Del Monte)	4.2	9
Grapefruit	4.2	3
Grapes	4.2	8
Kiwifruit	4.2	6
Lychee, canned in syrup and drained	4.2	16
Mango	4.2	8
Melon/cantaloupe	4.2	4
Oranges	4.2	5
Papaya	4.2	10
Peaches (raw or canned in natural juice)	4.2	5
Pear	4.2	4
Pineapple	4.2	7
Plum	4.2	5
Prunes, pitted	2.1	10
Raisins	2.1	28
Raspberries	4.2	1
Strawberries	4.2	1
Watermelon	4.2	4
Spreads		
Apricot fruit spread, reduced sugar	1.1	7
Blueberry spread (no sugar)	1.1	4
Hummus, purchased	1.1	1.5
Orange marmalade	1.1	9
Peanut butter (no sugar)	0.6	1
Pumpkinseed butter	0.6	1
Strawberry jam	1.1	10

(continued)

Glycemic Load of Common Foods, continued

Item	Serving size (in oz)	GL per serving
Snacks		
Cashews, salted	1.8	3
Chips, corn, plain, salted	1.8	17
Chips, potato, plain, salted	1.8	11
Olives, in brine	1.8	1
Peanuts	1.8	1
Popcorn, salted, no sugar	0.7	8
Pretzels, oven-baked, traditional	1.1	16
Vegetables		
Asparagus	4.4	2
Avocado	6.7	1
Beets	2.8	5
Broccoli	3.5	2
Carrots	2.8	3
Corn	2.8	9
Fava beans	2.8	9
Green beans	2.6	1
Green peas	2.8	3
Kale	2.6	1
Onion	6.3	2
Parsnips	2.8	12
Plantain, green	4.2	8
Potato, baked, without added fat	5.3	26
Potato, boiled	5.3	14
Potato, microwaved	5.3	14
Potato, new, unpeeled and boiled	5.3	16
Potato, white, baked in skin	5.3	18
Potatoes, french fried	5.3	22
Potatoes, instant mashed	5.3	17
Potatoes, mashed	5.3	15
Pumpkin	2.8	3

Item	Serving size (in oz)	GL per serving
Rutabaga	5.3	7
Sweet potato	5.3	17
Tomato	2.5	2
Yam	5.3	13
Desserts		
Apricot fruit bar (dried apricot filling in whole wheat pastry)	1.8	17
Chocolate bar, milk, plain	1.8	14
Jelly beans, assorted colors	1.1	22
Mars bar	2.1	26
Muesli bar containing dried fruit	1.1	13
Snickers	2.1	19
Twix	2.1	17

Source: The GL values of foods listed here are derived from research published by K. Foster-Powell, S. H. Holt, and J. C. Brand-Miller, "International Table of Glycemic Index and Glycemic Load Values," *American Journal of Clinical Nutrition* 76, no. 1 (2002): 5–56.

A comprehensive list of the GL of foods is available in *The New Optimum Nutrition Bible* and *The Holford Low-GL Diet*, or online at www.holforddiet.com.

HOW TO KEEP YOUR CHILD IN PERFECT BALANCE

As you can see abundantly in the chart above, the GL of some foods is through the roof and bound to play havoc with your child's blood sugar balance. You may have had a few shocks: baguettes and bagels have quite a high GL, for instance. But as you'll discover, it's amazingly easy to find thoroughly satisfying substitutes. Here are some examples of what your child should and should not be eating to keep her blood glucose level and brain in good balance:

INSTEAD OF	EAT
White toast and jelly	Whole-grain toast and unsweetened peanut butter
Sweetened cornflakes	Oatmeal with raspberries
Croissants and baguettes	Whole-grain rye breads

INSTEAD OF	EAT
White rice	Whole-grain spaghetti
Candy bars	Raw vegetable sticks
Bananas	Berries, apples, or oranges
Crackers or rice cakes	Oatcake crackers

Part 4 shows you how to do this in more detail. Now, let's look at what should be on your child's plate and what needs to stay on the supermarket shelves.

Sugar—The Long Goodbye

Weaning your child off sugar is a big part of the switch to brain-friendly eating. It's easiest for all concerned to decrease the sugar content of your child's diet slowly and gradually, so that she will get used to less sweetness without noticing it too much.

For example, sweeten cereal with fruit. Dilute fruit juices with water by at least half to halve their GL score (see page 28 for more advice on juices). Avoid foods with added sugar. Limit dried fruit, and cut down on fast-releasing, high-GL fruits like bananas, or combine them with slow-releasing, low-GL carbohydrates such as oat cereals.

The one exception to this rule is when your child has just done some intense exercise, such as playing a game of hockey. She'll need to boost her blood sugar levels fast, as not only are her blood sugar levels low, but the glycogen storage facilities in her muscles and liver will also be empty. So there is no harm in her snacking on a fast-releasing fruit such as a banana: any excess glucose in the blood will go to replenish the empty glycogen storage facilities rather than build up into high blood sugar.

Stay Away from Sugar Substitutes

While they won't raise blood sugar levels, sugar substitutes shouldn't be part of your plan to cut down on sugar in your child's diet. Aspartame, the most widely used, is particularly bad. Plenty of studies have shown it to have adverse effects on health in children. One study into the effects of aspartame showed that it caused nightmares, memory loss, temper, and nausea.[6] Besides the dangers of additives, there is another good reason not to use them: they don't help children adjust to less sweet food. For all of us, adults and children alike, staying away from sugar becomes easier and easier as our cravings for sugar subside. Artificial sweeteners simply keep those cravings alive.

There are two sugar substitutes that are worth a mention. The first is agave nectar. This sweetener is derived from the agave cactus and is gaining in popularity. While it is derived from a natural source and is low GL, its high fructose content is cause for caution. Fructose occurs naturally in fruit; however, high consumption of processed fructose has been linked with worse levels of blood fats such as cholesterol and triglycerides. These are the sort of blood fat profiles seen in older people with heart disease, obesity, and diabetes. The second sweetener to mention is xylitol. It is derived from a natural source and is abundant in plums, which have a very low GL as a result. Xylitol has a fraction of the effect on blood sugar compared with regular sugar or even fructose. For example, 9 teaspoons of xylitol has the same effect on the blood sugar as 4 teaspoons of fructose or 1 teaspoon of sugar. Regardless, we still suggest you reduce your child's taste for sweet foods, but when some sweetness is really essential, for example, if you're whipping up dessert for a special-occasion meal, then xylitol is the best alternative to sugar.

Dynamic Duo—Protein and Fiber

The more fiber and protein you include with any meal or snack, the slower the release of the carbohydrates. Fiber does the job by actually getting in the way of the carbohydrate, impeding its interaction with digestive enzymes and effectively slowing its passage into the intestines, where it is absorbed into the bloodstream. Meanwhile, protein slows down the speed at which the stomach empties its contents of partially digested food into the intestines.

As we've seen, anything that slows the passage of carbohydrate into the bloodstream is good for blood glucose balance. So combining protein-rich foods with high-fiber carbohydrates is an excellent rule of thumb in this context. Here's how you do it:

- Give seeds or nuts with a fruit snack.
- Add seeds or nuts to carbohydrate-based breakfast cereals.
- Serve fish, chicken, or tofu with brown basmati rice.

- Add kidney beans to sauce served over whole-grain pasta.
- Put cottage cheese on oatcake crackers, or hummus on rye bread.
- Make sandwiches with unsweetened peanut butter and whole-grain bread.

Is It Really Juice?

Much of the so-called fruit juice on the market is not much better than sugary water. Once a fruit juice has been processed and put into a carton, it bears little resemblance to a fresh fruit juice in terms of color, taste, and nutrient content.

Unfortunately, however, the sugar content remains intact. Children who regularly drink processed juice are taking in a lot of sugar and thereby messing up their blood glucose balance, feeding their sugar cravings, and rotting their teeth. Despite vigorous marketing to convince us to the contrary, the stuff in these cartons is not a good source of vitamins and minerals. Worst of all are the "juice drinks"—these almost invariably have added sugars and very little actual fruit juice.

This doesn't mean juice is completely off the menu. You simply need to go for freshly squeezed, or failing that, refrigerated juices, which are obviously fresher; just be vigilant about checking labels to discover its shelf life. If this is longer than just a few days into the future, we recommend you don't touch it. If it is expected to go bad in a few days, then it was probably reasonably nutritious when it went into the carton, but its nutrient content is declining by the hour. So inevitably, fruit that's juiced right in front of you is the best bet.

Along with freshness, you need to look at the GL score of various juices. Apple and pear are best, followed by orange. As we mentioned above, it's also important to dilute the juice your child drinks by at least half, with water, as this halves the GL score. Fresh vegetable juices can be drunk without dilution, with the possible exception of carrot juice.

Don't Go without Breakfast

Getting your child up on a school morning with enough time for her to eat a decent breakfast can be challenging at the best of times. But eating a decent breakfast really is essential for your child to be able to concentrate in school. If her blood sugar stays at rock-bottom all morning, she'll experience all the problems we've mentioned, from dizziness to a lack of mental focus.

In one study, twenty-nine schoolchildren were given different breakfast cereals, a glucose drink, or no breakfast, on different days. Their attention and memory were tested before breakfast and again 30, 90, 150, and 210 minutes later. Children who had had the glucose drink or no breakfast showed poorer attention and memory compared to the children eating cereal.[7]

We find that children who eat a nutritious diet generally get a much better night's sleep, too (see chapter 20). Consequently, it's easier for them to get out of bed in the morning, which in turn gives them the time and inclination to eat a decent breakfast.

If your child doesn't have much of an appetite in the morning and frequently skips breakfast, help her by easing her into the habit gradually. Begin by giving her one strawberry. The next day, make it two strawberries and a Brazil nut or a teaspoon of sunflower seeds. The next day, provide half an apple and three almonds, and so on, until after a couple of weeks she'll be able to eat a bowl of oatmeal with fruit and nuts. Remember that you too need to eat breakfast! If you typically go to work on a cup of coffee, don't be surprised if your children attempt to imitate you in their own way.

Stay Off the Caffeine

Sugar isn't the only factor in blood sugar problems. Stimulants are, too, and as caffeine is a powerful one, it can be highly disruptive to your child's blood sugar balance. Caffeine is also an appetite suppressant, and as such can be implicated in behaviors like picky eating or refusing to contemplate breakfast.

Supermarket shelves groan with products containing caffeine. Let's look at the biggest culprits.

COLA AND ENERGY DRINKS

Colas and energy drinks contain anything from 46 to 80 mg of caffeine per can, as much as you'd find in a cup of filtered coffee. These drinks are often also high in sugar and colorings, and their net stimulant effect can be considerable. Check the label on all canned drinks, and keep your children away from any that contain caffeine and chemical additives or colorings. Also watch out for "natural" stimulants like guarana: these have the same effect as caffeine.

CANDY BARS AND DRINKS

Candy bars and chocolates are everywhere these days, along with hordes of sugarholics. The bars are usually full of sugar, which is bad enough for blood glucose levels, but cocoa, the active ingredient in chocolate and chocolate drinks, also provides significant quantities of the stimulant theobromine. Theobromine's action is similar to caffeine's, though not as strong. Chocolate also contains small amounts of caffeine.

As chocolate is high in sugar and stimulants, reserve it as a special treat for your child. That means a small amount once a week rather than every day. Also bear in mind the relative size of the candy bar and your child. For example, don't give a toddler more than a small piece of candy at one sitting.

COFFEE AND TEA

Coffee consumption is increasing, particularly among teens, who tend to hang out in the ubiquitous coffee shops of the modern age. Coffee contains three stimulants: caffeine, theobromine, and theophylline. Although caffeine is the strongest of the three, theophylline is known to disturb normal sleep patterns and theobromine has a similar effect to caffeine's, although it is present in much smaller amounts in coffee. Decaffeinated coffee isn't stimulant free, because only some of the caffeine is removed and the other stimulants remain. Tea is only slightly better than coffee; a strong cup of tea can contain as much caffeine as a weak cup of coffee and is certainly addictive. Tea also contains tannin, which interferes with the absorption of vital minerals such as iron and zinc. Even decaffeinated tea is not actually caffeine free; it simply has reduced caffeine and the same tannin levels.

So there's a host of stimulants in coffee waiting to mess up your teenager's blood sugar balance. But that's not all. It is also addictive, and despite general public perception, it actually worsens mental performance. Research published in the *American Journal of Psychiatry* studied 1,500 psychology students and found that moderate and high consumers of coffee have higher levels of anxiety and depression than abstainers and that the high consumers had the greatest incidence of stress-related medical problems, as well as lower academic performance.[8] A number of studies have shown that the ability to remember lists of words is made worse by caffeine, so children who drink coffee before school, especially as a pre-exam boost, are more likely to struggle in class.

The reason people get hooked on caffeine, particularly in the morning, is that it makes you feel better, more energized, and alert. However, Dr. Peter Rogers, a psychologist at Bristol University, wondered whether caffeine actually increases your energy and mental performance or just relieves the symptoms of withdrawal.

When he researched this, he found that, after that sacred cup of coffee, coffee drinkers don't feel any better than people who never drink coffee—they just feel better than they did when they woke up.[9] In other words, drinking coffee relieves the symptoms of withdrawal from caffeine. So the important message here is, don't let your child start drinking coffee. It isn't good for her, and like any addiction, giving up it becomes more difficult the longer you have the habit.

If you want to give your child a hot drink, the most popular alternatives are Teeccino, Pero, or Bambu (made with roasted chicory and malted barley), or herb teas. You will find the coffee alternatives at health food stores, some grocery stores, or online. Herb teas are more widely available, and you should find them in good supermarkets too. If your child already has a taste for coffee, offer a choice of these substitutes. She may experience withdrawal symptoms when she gives up coffee, such as headaches, but these will disappear within a few days.

In summary, here are some general guidelines to ensure your child's brain gets an even supply of glucose:

- Choose whole foods—whole grains, lentils, beans, nuts, seeds, fresh fruit, and vegetables. With fruits and vegetables, go for dark green, leafy, and root vegetables such as spinach, carrots, yams, broccoli, Brussels sprouts, green beans, or bell peppers, raw or lightly cooked. Choose fresh fruits such as apples, pears, berries, cantaloupe, or citrus fruits and, infrequently, bananas. Provide five or more servings of fruits and vegetables each day.

- Avoid overly processed foods.
- Choose whole grains such as rice, buckwheat, millet, rye, oats, whole wheat, corn, or quinoa in cereal, breads, and pasta. Avoid refined "white" foods.
- Avoid sugar and foods containing sugar, meaning anything with added corn syrup, maple syrup, glucose, sucrose, or dextrose. Keep fructose consumption within limits. Don't be tempted to go for sugar substitutes—most are detrimental to health and they all keep sugar cravings alive.
- Combine protein foods with carbohydrate foods by giving cereals and fruit with nuts or seeds and ensuring your child eats carbohydrate-rich foods such as potatoes, bread, pasta, or rice with protein-rich foods such as fish, chicken, lentils, beans, or tofu. As fiber is important for slowing sugar absorption, make sure your child is getting ample fiber in fruits and vegetables.
- Choose real, fresh fruit juices from the refrigerated case and dilute by at least half. Avoid the highly processed kind with a long shelf life.
- Encourage your child to eat breakfast.
- Help your child avoid caffeinated food and drinks, such as chocolate and sodas.

Chapter 3

Smart Fats— The Mind's Construction Crew

We humans are fatheaded: the solid part of our brains is a good 60 percent fat. In a child, this fatty tissue is constantly growing and maintaining itself, so a good supply of the raw materials—essential fats—is needed to build a healthy brain. These aren't just any old fats, and it's vital that your child gets the right kind, in the right quantities.

Three-year-old Adrian is a case in point. His parents brought him to see us at the Brain Bio Centre because they were concerned about his loss of speech development. They had already put him on a dairy- and gluten-free diet and were pleased to see that his eczema disappeared and his asthma had improved dramatically. We ran some tests that showed he was very low in magnesium, selenium, and zinc and also in essential fats. We recommended supplementation of fish oils and a multivitamin and mineral formula. Within days of starting the fish oil, Adrian began to chatter again.

Check your child out on the questionnaire below.

Fat Check

Does your child:

- ❏ Eat oily fish (salmon, trout, sardines, herring, mackerel, or fresh tuna) less than once a week?
- ❏ Eat seeds or their cold-pressed oils fewer than three times a week?
- ❏ Eat meat or dairy products most days?
- ❏ Eat processed or fried foods (such as ready-to-eat meals, french fries, or potato chips) three or more times a week?
- ❏ Have dry or rough skin or a tendency to eczema?
- ❏ Have dry or dull hair or dandruff?
- ❏ Suffer from dry, watery, or itchy eyes?
- ❏ Suffer from excessive thirst or frequent urination?
- ❏ Have frequent mood swings?
- ❏ Have a poor memory, short attention span, or difficulty concentrating?
- ❏ Have poor physical coordination?

Check the box for each "yes" answer. If you check five or more, the chances are your child isn't getting enough essential fats. By upping your child's intake, these symptoms can rapidly improve.

We'll be explaining later in this chapter how to dramatically boost your child's essential fat levels with the right food and supplements. But first, let's look more closely at what they do.

ESSENTIAL FATS—MIRACLE IN MIND

Essential fats—the omega-3 and omega-6 essential fats—help children stay physically healthy, reducing the risk of allergies, asthma, eczema, and infections. More than this, they promote mental health. A deficiency can result in depression, dyslexia, attention deficit disorder, autism, fatigue, and memory and behavior problems. The bottom line is that essential fats really *are* essential for keeping the state of your child's brain in healthy equilibrium. And these fats are also needed in optimal amounts to maximize your child's intelligence.

We use the word "intelligence" very broadly here. Your child's ability to perform in this world depends upon a balance of mental, emotional, and physical intelligence. Mental intelligence we are very well aware of, because of IQ tests that determine a person's ability to make intellectual connections and deal with complex concepts.

But emotional intelligence is no less important. Your child's EQ is a measure of his ability to respond emotionally to situations in an appropriate and sensitive way. If he loses his temper easily and oscillates between depression and hyperactivity, lacking emotional balance and perspective, there's room for improvement—however bright he may be.

Then there's physical intelligence. PQ is all about brain-body coordination. For example, a lot of children diagnosed with attention deficit disorder are clumsy by nature (with or without a diagnosis of dyspraxia, a learning disorder that affects coordination) and have trouble with skills such as handwriting, reading, and taking notes in class.

Never Too Late to Start

Every type of intelligence—IQ, EQ, and PQ—is affected by your child's intake of the omega-3s and omega-6s. Children deficient in essential fats have more learning difficulties, while children who were breast-fed have higher IQs at age eight than those who were bottle-fed, which is thought to be due to the higher levels of essential fats in breast milk.[1]

Recent studies by Dr. Peter Willatts at the University of Dundee in Scotland showed that babies fed a formula enriched with a specific essential fat (DHA) had better problem-solving skills at ten months of age.[2] Also, supplementation of omega-3 essential fats to women while pregnant and breast-feeding has been shown to improve their child's intellectual function right up to their fourth year.[3] Research underway is likely to show that these benefits persist into adulthood.

Essential fats remain essentially important throughout life, so your child will continue to need them as he grows, and beyond. The good news is that it's never too late to boost your child's essential fat levels so that he can reap the benefits.

For example, research by Dr. Alex Richardson at Oxford University has proven the value of essential fats in a double-blind trial involving forty-one children aged eight to twelve years who had symptoms of attention deficit/hyperactivity disorder (ADHD) and specific learning difficulties. Since the study was double-blind, no one involved knew who was getting the essential fats and who was getting the placebo until the trail was over and the results analyzed, thus avoiding bias in both the scientists and the children. The children who received extra essential fats in supplements were both behaving and learning better within twelve weeks.[4] Another trial by Dr. Richardson showed significant improvement in reading ability in children on essential fat supplements, compared with children taking a placebo, over six months.[5]

All this confirms surveys carried out at Purdue University that show children with ADHD tend to get lower levels of essential fats than children without ADHD.[6] Supplementation with these was found to reduce ADHD symptoms such as anxiety, attention difficulties, and general behavior problems.[7]

So, while it seems such a simple thing, giving your child an essential fat supplement can have profound benefits for his mental abilities.

How Omegas Do the Job

All the evidence points to essential fats as vital to the ongoing task of keeping your child in good mental health. In fact, the brain and nervous system totally depend on them, and never more so than during pregnancy and childhood. The other important fat families are saturated and monounsaturated fats and cholesterol. Your child's brain contains vast amounts of cholesterol, for instance, and it is used to make the sex hormones estrogen, progesterone, and testosterone. But these fats can be made in the body. The omega fats have to be supplied through diet, which is why you need to ensure your child's level of them stays topped up.

To fully understand what omega fats do in the brain, let's take a closer look at a neuron.

As we saw in chapter 1, intelligence—and the process of thought itself—involves the careful connecting up of billions of nerve cells, each one of which links to thousands of others. You'll remember that the "messengers," neurotransmitters, deliver their messages across connection points called synapses into receptor sites.

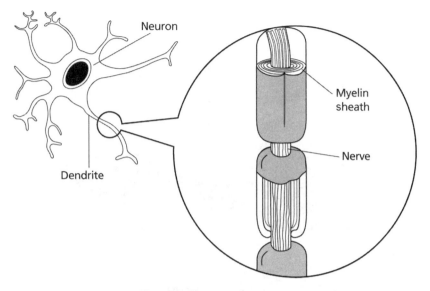

Figure 5. Close-up of a neuron

These receptor sites are contained within the myelin sheath, which surrounds every neuron in the brain. The sheath is a bit like a layer of insulation around an electrical wire. Without it, the transmission of messages—and thus, the working of the brain—would be impossible. The sheath is roughly 75 percent fat, and it's here that the omegas have a starring role.

Myelin sheath fat is made out of phospholipids (more on these in the next chapter), each with a saturated and unsaturated fatty acid attached. In figure 6 you'll see the unsaturated fatty acid as a bent squiggle, which is most often an omega-3 or omega-6 fat.

Both kinds of omega fats need to be in balance—in fact, this balance seems to be critical for the smooth working and restructuring of the brain. So for brain health, you'll need to supply both omega-3 and omega-6 fats in your child's diet.

OMEGA-3 AND OMEGA-6 IN YOUR CHILD'S DIET

Despite all the evidence in favor of essential fats, many adults and increasingly more children are fat-phobic and may shy away from taking them. The reason is that all types of fat are generally lumped together and fat gets a lot of bad press.

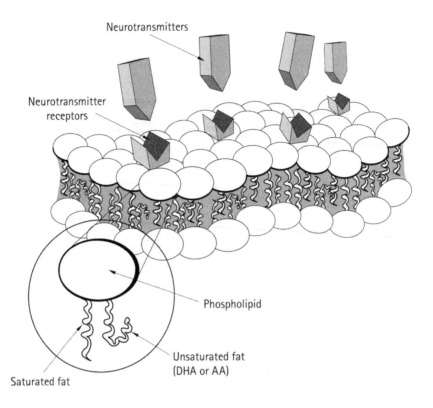

Figure 6. The myelin sheath surrounding neurons,
composed of phospholipids and fats

Some of this is deserved. The damaged or hydrogenated (solidified) fats found in processed or fried foods and some margarines are bad for health, yet they're everywhere, as are saturated fats in dairy products and meat. As a result, most people in the United States are eating too much of them.

But this doesn't mean you need to put your child on a low-fat diet. You just need to ensure that the fats in his diet are the right kind—the omegas. If your child is concerned that eating them will lead to weight gain, you should know that they can actually help with weight loss! So even if your child is overweight, he should still be eating essential fats, while cutting down on the saturated fats in meat and dairy, and completely cutting out the trans fats found in fried and processed foods. (Chapter 23 will tell you what to look for on labels to avoid these fats.)

Most of us are deficient in the omega fats, particularly in omega-3s, as we will see. And many children are grossly deficient, as the many child health problems related to deficiency show. Ultimately, however, the most precise way to know your child's essential fat status is to have a blood test. We give a blood test at our London-based Brain Bio Centre, and the test is also available through nutritionists. The test gives you a complete breakdown of all the essential fats and which ones are lacking.

Fat Figures

How much essential fat will your child need to stay mentally and physically healthy? To answer that, we first need to look at the optimal amount of overall fat in his diet.

It is best to consume no more than 20 percent of all calories as fat. The current average in the United States is around 40 percent. In countries with a low incidence of fat-related diseases such as heart disease, like Japan, Thailand, and the Philippines, people consume only about 15 percent of their total calorie intake from fat.

Most authorities now agree that of our total fat intake, no more than one-third should be saturated fat, and at least one-third should be polyunsaturated oils providing the two essential fats, omega-3 and omega-6. As

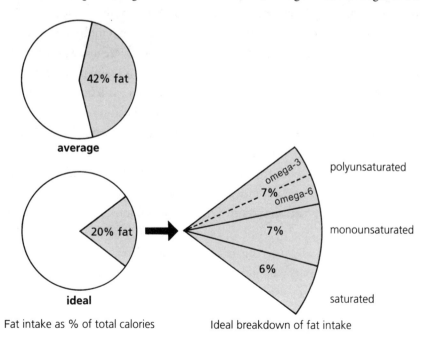

Figure 7. What we eat versus what we need

we saw earlier, these two essential fat families also need to be roughly in balance—in a ratio of 1:1, which is what our ancestors were getting before the Industrial Revolution. Then, people ate local foods with an abundance of seeds, whereas the widespread exodus to the cities resulted in the rise of easily stored refined foods and hard fats. So nowadays, the average balance is more like 1:20 in favor of omega-6s.

So it may not be just the gross deficiency in omega-3 fats that has led to so many of the health problems we're seeing in children today, but also the gross imbalance between the two omegas. In addition, a high intake of saturated fats and the damaged polyunsaturated fats we call trans fats stop the body from making good use of the little essential fat the average person does eat in a day.

The Omega-3s

By now, you'll have gathered how important the omega fat families are to your child's mental and emotional health. Let's delve more deeply, first taking a closer look at the essential fats so many children lack—the omega-3s.

Why is the modern-day diet likely to be more deficient in omega-3 fats than in omega-6s? It's all because the grandmother of the omega-3 family, alpha-linolenic acid, and her metabolically active grandchildren EPA (eicosapentaenoic acid) and DHA (docosahexaenoic acid), are more unsaturated and so more prone to damage by cooking, heating, and food processing. For example, if you fry a piece of fish or roast seeds, you will actually damage some of the omega-3s they contain. In any event, the average person today eats a mere sixth of the omega-3 fats found in the average diet of 1850. This decline is partly due to food choices, but mainly due to food processing.

Alpha-linolenic acid, the omega-3 grandmother, is abundant in cold climate seeds, such as flaxseeds, and also plankton, the vegetation of the sea. Our bodies can convert some of this alpha-linolenic acid into EPA and DHA, but a more effective way to increase supplies of these more active omega-3s is to eat oily fish; this is because the fish has already effectively done the conversion for us in its own body. The primary source of EPA and DHA is coldwater fish, especially fish that eat fish—namely herring, mackerel, salmon, and fresh tuna. Sardines are also an excellent source.

There are a few caveats here. Since canned tuna has much less omega-3, stick with fresh tuna. But as larger fish like tuna tend to be higher in mer-

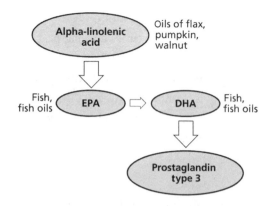

Figure 8. Omega-3 fat family

cury, don't feed tuna steaks to your child more than once a week, and less if he shows signs of mercury toxicity (more on this in chapter 7). As for salmon, the amount of EPA and DHA in farmed fish really depends on the quality of their diet, and as with most intensive farming practices, this can be variable. Organic farmed or wild salmon is much better in this respect.

As a rule of thumb, children normally need around 300 to 400 mg of both DHA and EPA a day (see chapter 26 for supplement levels for different age ranges). The conversion in the body of alpha-linolenic acid in, say, flaxseeds and pumpkinseeds to EPA and DHA can be very inefficient. For this reason, vegetarians rarely have sufficient levels of EPA and DHA unless they eat significant quantities of flaxseeds, which are the richest source of alpha-linolenic acid.

So during critical periods of development such as childhood, it may be preferable to get a direct source of EPA and DHA from fish, backed up by an indirect supply from flaxseeds or flaxseed oil; this would certainly be recommended for a pregnant or breast-feeding woman to allow her to pass on sufficient EPA and DHA to her child. The World Health Organization now recommends that infant formulas include these oils.[8] DHA is especially important during the fetal stage and infancy because it is literally used to build the brain and makes up a full quarter of the brain's dry weight.

In many cases, children with learning and behavioral problems are even less efficient than average at converting alpha-linolenic acid into EPA and DHA. Partly for this reason, a child with ADHD or dyslexia may need to take double or triple the recommended amount to correct his condition.

The best diet from the point of view of omega-3 fats is a "fishitarian" one where your child eats fish three times a week; or, failing that, a seed-rich vegan diet. Eggs can also provide significant quantities of omega-3 if the hens were fed a high-omega-3 diet—check the egg carton labels.

Remember: Not only is it important to eat a direct source of omega-3 fats such as fish or a rich, indirect source such as flaxseeds, it's also vital for your child to eat less saturated and processed fat. We'll see why in a bit.

The Omega-6s

Your child will also need omega-6 fats. Of all the tissues of the body, the brain has the highest proportion of these fats.

The grandmother of the omega-6 fat family is linoleic acid, which is found in hot-climate seeds such as sunflower and sesame seeds. Linoleic acid is converted by the body into gamma-linolenic acid (GLA), which may be familiar to you as a substance in evening primrose oil and borage or starflower oil, the richest known sources. A derivative of GLA, known as DGLA, is found in high quantities in the brain.

Supplementing GLA, usually from evening primrose oil, has proven effective in alleviating a wide variety of mental health problems. For example, a study on children with dyspraxia showed that supplementation with essential fats including omega-6 oil improved reading, writing, and behavior in just three months.[9]

One omega-6 fat has something of a Jekyll and Hyde nature, however, and that's arachidonic acid (AA). While there is no question that it is essential for brain function, arachidonic acid is bad news in excess in the body, as it is

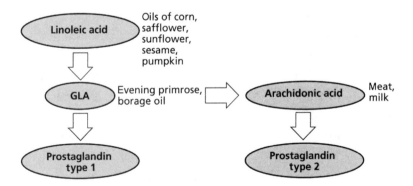

Figure 9. Omega-6 fat family

associated with promoting inflammation. It can be derived either directly from meat or animal products, or indirectly from linoleic acid or GLA. The latter may be a preferable source because GLA also produces anti-inflammatory substances (type 1 prostaglandins) that balance the inflammatory effects of the type 2 prostaglandins made from arachidonic acid. (The type 3 prostaglandins made from omega-3 fatty acids are also anti-inflammatory.)

For this and other reasons, it's best to let your child eat omega-6-rich seeds and their oils to get enough of this essential fat family, rather than overdosing on meat and dairy products.

Where to Get the Omegas

As we've seen, the seeds with the highest levels of omega-3 fats are flaxseeds. Hempseeds and pumpkinseeds are rich sources, too. The only direct source of the essential omega-3 brain boosters EPA and DHA are oily fish.

The best seeds for omega-6 fats are hemp, pumpkin, sunflower, safflower, and sesame, and corn kernels. Walnuts, soybeans, and wheat germ are also rich in omega-6s.

Best Foods for Brain Fats

OMEGA-3	OMEGA-6	EPA & DHA	GLA
Flaxseeed	Corn oil	Salmon	Evening primrose oil
Hempseeds	Safflower oil	Mackerel	
Pumpkinseeds	Sesame	Herring	Borage or starflower oil
	Sunflower	Sardines	
	Walnut	Anchovies (whole, not salted fillets)	Black currant seed oil
		Tuna steak	
		Eggs (of flaxseed-fed hens)	

So what's the best way to incorporate these essential fats into your child's daily menu? There are three possibilities: seeds and fish; seed oils, which are more concentrated in essential fats but don't provide other nutrients such as minerals, which are abundant in the whole seeds; or supplementing concentrated fish oils and seed oils such as flax, evening primrose, or borage oil.

Now let's look at how to put those ideas into practice.

SEEDS AND FISH

If you want to go with seeds, put one measure each of sesame seeds, sunflower seeds, and pumpkinseeds, and three measures of flaxseeds, into a sealed jar. Keep it in the fridge, away from light, heat, and oxygen. Simply adding 1 heaping tablespoon of these seeds, freshly ground in a coffee grinder, to your child's breakfast each morning guarantees a good daily intake of essential fats. We'd also recommend that your child eats 3.5 ounces (100 g) of oily fish (roughly equivalent in size to one tin of sardines or a salmon fillet) two or three times a week.

SEED OILS

If you want to use oils, the best place to start is an oil blend that offers a 1:1 ratio of omega-3 and omega-6 fats and is cold-pressed, preferably organic, and kept refrigerated before you buy it. These are now widely available in health food stores. The oil can be added to salads and other cold or warm foods but must not be heated. Some children will eat it straight off the spoon.

Hempseed oil is the next best thing. It provides 19 percent alpha-linolenic acid (omega-3), 57 percent linoleic acid (omega-6), and 2 percent GLA (omega-6). Chapter 26 gives details of supplement levels for different age ranges.

SUPPLEMENTS

As far as supplements are concerned, for omega-6 your best bet is borage oil or evening primrose oil. Borage oil provides more GLA, and fish oils are best for omega-3. There are supplements that combine EPA, DHA, and GLA. For smaller children who can't swallow supplements, there are a number of supplements in liquid form and flavored in various ways. Levels of these to supplement are discussed in detail in chapter 26.

FATS TO AVOID OR LIMIT

The kind of fat your child eats alters the fat composition in his brain. If it's the omega or other fats that were there in the first place, all is well; but if it's the fats that so much junk and other processed foods are riddled with, your child will be rebuilding his brain with fats that fail to manage the brainwork required of him.

Trans Fat—The Worst Culprit

The worst fats your child can eat are the trans fats we've talked about— damaged fats found in deep-fried food and foods containing hydrogenated vegetable oils. To minimize your child's exposure to trans fats, limit his intake of fried and especially deep-fried food and don't buy foods containing hydrogenated fats. Check the list of ingredients in processed foods: if a food has the word "hydrogenated" in the ingredients, don't put it in your basket. Another clue is shelf life. Trans fats are widely used to extend shelf life, so a long shelf life is a warning sign that the food probably contains trans fats and/or preservatives.

Why are trans fats so bad for your child? They can be taken directly into the brain and appear in the same position as DHA in brain cells, where they proceed to make a hash of the information-processing job DHA does so brilliantly. Trans fats also block the conversion of essential fats into vital brain fats such as GLA and DHA. Twice as many trans fats appear in the brains of people deficient in omega-3 fats.

So a combined deficiency in omega-3 fats and an excess of trans fats— the hallmark of the chicken-nugget-and-fries generation—is a bad scenario. A serving of french fries or fried fish can each deliver 8 g of trans fats, a doughnut 12 g, and a bag of chips more than 4 g. Fortunately, since 2006, the FDA requires trans fats to be declared on labels, making them much easier to spot. The ideal amount in your child's diet is zero.

Saturated and Monounsaturated Fats

Saturated fats are typically solid at room temperature and include butter, cheese, lard (the fat in meat), and coconut oil. While you don't want your child to eat large amounts of saturated fat, a small amount is fine. One good use of these fats is for frying. Saturated fats are not damaged by heat and converted into trans fats in the way that the polyunsaturated fats such as the omega fats are. So we suggest using butter or virgin coconut oil if you're frying food at home. Always fry at the lowest possible temperature to reduce the amount of oxidants you create (more on this in chapter 6).

Monounsaturated fats, which include olive oil, are liquid at room temperature but will start solidifying if refrigerated (the omega fats and other polyunsaturated fats remain liquid even at much lower temperatures). There is plenty of research to show that good-quality olive oil contributes to health. Extra-virgin olive oil is ideal for raw use such as in salad dressings but is not suitable for frying, as it is more susceptible to damage from heat. If you want to fry with olive oil, use medium or mild varieties, as these are more robust, and keep the heat low.

Cholesterol

Similar to saturated fats, a moderate amount of cholesterol in the diet is perfectly acceptable and even necessary. How good or bad it is depends on how it's cooked. Overcooked, fried, or burned cholesterol is bad for your child's health, so don't fry eggs or bacon until they are crisp, or char meat.

> **In summary, here are some general guidelines to ensure your child gets enough brain fats:**
>
> - Provide plenty of seeds and nuts—the best seeds are flax, hemp, pumpkin, sunflower, and sesame. You get more goodness out of them by grinding them first and sprinkling on cereal, soups, and salads.
> - Choose coldwater carnivorous fish—a serving of sardines, herring, or wild/organic salmon two or three times a week provides a good source of omega-3 fats. Choose larger oily fish such as tuna, swordfish, or king mackerel less often due to the high mercury content.
> - Choose cold-pressed seed oils—either an oil blend or hempseed oil—for salad dressings and other cold uses.
> - Avoid fried food and processed food.
> - Choose fish oil to supplement omega-3 fats, and borage or evening primrose oil for omega-6 fats.

Chapter 4

Phospholipids—
Go to School
on an Egg

Phospholipids are the "intelligent" fats in our brains. They are rather complicated conglomerations that include phosphorous (phospho-) and fatty acids (-lipids), hence their name. They are a major component of membranes of every single cell in the body as well as being the insulation experts, helping make up the myelin sheath that covers all nerves, and promoting a smooth run for all the signals in the brain. Phospholipids—found in fish (especially sardines), eggs, organ meats, soy-derived lecithin, and other foods—make the brain sing, enhancing your child's mood, mind, and mental performance.

Check your child out on the questionnaire below.

Phospholipid Check

Does your child:

- ❏ Eat fish less than once a week?
- ❏ Eat fewer than three eggs per week?
- ❏ Eat soy/tofu or nuts less than three times per week?
- ❏ Take less than 5 g of lecithin each day?
- ❏ Have a poor memory?
- ❏ Find it hard to do calculations in her head?
- ❏ Sometimes have difficulty concentrating?

❑ Have a tendency toward depression?
❑ Appear to be a slow learner?

Check the box for each "yes" answer. If you check five or more, the chances are your child isn't getting enough phospholipids.

SUPERBRAINS IN THE MAKING?

There are two kinds of phospholipids: phosphatidylcholine and phosphatidylserine, otherwise known as PC and PS. Supplementing these smart fats, as well as eating foods rich in choline and serine, from which they're built, has some very positive benefits for your child's brain. Let's look at choline first.

Choline—Memories Are Made of This

To give you some idea of just how dramatic the effect of choline on the brain can be, consider this study from the Duke University Medical Center. During it, researchers demonstrated that giving choline during pregnancy creates the equivalent of superbrains in rat offspring.

The team fed choline to female rats halfway through their pregnancy. The infant rats whose mothers had been fed the choline had vastly superior brains with more neuronal connections and, consequently, improved learning ability and better memory recall, all of which persisted into old age. In essence, this research shows that giving choline helps restructure the brain for improved performance.[1] And although the focus was on rats, we would expect a similar effect in humans.

Choline is a star performer in mental ability because it is the direct source of acetylcholine, the memory neurotransmitter in our brains. In fact, choline deficiency is a common cause for poor memory.

Supplementing choline not only makes more acetylcholine.[2] It also forms a vital building material for nerve cells and the receptor sites for neurotransmitters. According to Professor Richard Wurtman of the Massachusetts Institute of Technology, if your choline levels are depleted, your body grabs the choline that you need to build your nerve cells to make more acetylcholine.[3] So Wurtman believes that providing the brain with enough of this vital brain nutrient is essential.

PS: Don't Forget the Phosphatidylserine

Phosphatidylserine, sometimes known as the memory molecule, is a smart nutrient that can genuinely boost your child's brainpower. The secret to the memory-boosting properties of PS is probably its ability to help brain cells communicate, as it is a vital part of the structure of the brain's receptor sites.

The positive effects of supplementing PS are just as amazing as those of supplementing choline. We've seen children with learning problems completely overcome them just by adding a source of these vital phospholipids.

EAT YOUR PHOSPHOLIPIDS

Although we can make phospholipids in the body, getting some extra from dietary sources is even better.

The richest sources of phospholipids in the average diet, as we've seen, are eggs and organ meats, which explains why lions and other animals at the top of the food chain eat the organs and brain first—they're not stupid! You can also find choline in soybeans, peanuts, and other nuts.

But nowadays, as the number of children suffering from memory and concentration problems soars, our intake of phospholipids is sinking dramatically. For example, to top up our dietary PS to the level of about 50 mg a day, we'd have to eat a lot of liver and other organ meats—not a very likely scenario these days. Vegetarians are unlikely to achieve even 10 mg of PS a day.

A daily supplement can really help some children's memories—see chapter 26 for details of amounts for different age ranges. Phospholipids are often a part of brain food formulas. And there are other ways of getting these wonder fats back into your child's diet—let's look at them now.

Rediscover the Egg

Eggs are delicious, as well as the richest source of choline and an excellent source of PS. But people these days are often egg-phobic, thinking that they are an unwholesome food due to their high fat and cholesterol content. This just isn't true. As we learned in the last chapter, some fat and cholesterol are essential for health.

The kind of fat you find in eggs depends on what you feed the chickens. If you feed them a diet rich in omega-3s, for example flaxseeds or fishmeal, you get an egg high in omega-3s. An egg is as healthful as the chicken that laid it.

As for cholesterol, it is simply a myth that what you find in eggs is bad for you or your child—it will neither raise blood cholesterol nor cause heart disease. And as long as you don't fry it, a free-range, organic, omega-3-rich egg is a veritable superfood. Go for lightly boiled or hardboiled eggs, or gently scramble them; you can safely give your child six to ten eggs a week.

Lecithin—Gold in Those Granules

Lecithin is the best source of phospholipids and is widely available in health food stores, where it's sold either as lecithin granules or capsules. The easiest and cheapest way to take this is to add a tablespoon of lecithin to your child's cereal in the morning.

And in case you were wondering, lecithin won't make your child fat. In fact, quite the opposite: it helps the body digest fat.

In summary, here are some general guidelines to help ensure your child has an optimal intake of phospholipids:

- Add a tablespoon of lecithin granules to your child's cereal every day.
- Or give your child an egg for breakfast, preferably free-range, organic, high in omega-3s, and lightly boiled or scrambled, but definitely not fried.
- Or supplement with a brain food formula providing phosphatidylcholine and phosphatidylserine, especially if your child is having learning problems.

Chapter 5

Protein—
The Architect of
Mind and Mood

Protein provides amino acids, the building blocks of life. Just as a sentence is made up of words and words of letters, protein is made up of peptides and peptides are made up of amino acids.

When your child eats protein-rich foods such as meat, eggs, fish, dairy, lentils, beans, or quinoa (a South American grain, pronounced "keen-wa"), her digestive system breaks down the protein first into peptides and then into amino acids. By linking amino acids together in different sequences, her body then builds up new muscle or organ tissue or neurotransmitters—the chemical messengers of the brain. So a good supply of protein, and hence of amino acids, will keep your child's brain running super-smoothly.

Deficiency in amino acids isn't at all uncommon and can give rise to depression, apathy and lack of motivation, inability to relax, poor memory, and concentration. But supplementing specific amino acids has been proven to correct all these problems. For example, a form of the amino acid tryptophan has proven more effective in double-blind trials than the best antidepressant drugs, the amino acid tyrosine improves mental and physical performance under stress better than coffee, and the amino acid GABA is highly effective against anxiety.[1]

Amino Acid Check

Does your child:

- ❏ Eat less than one portion of protein-rich foods (meat, dairy, fish, eggs, tofu) each day?
- ❏ Eat fewer than two servings of vegetable sources of protein (beans, lentils, quinoa, seeds, nuts, whole grains, and so on) each day?
- ❏ If she's vegetarian, does she rarely combine different protein foods such as those mentioned above?
- ❏ Engage in a lot of physical activity?
- ❏ Suffer from anxiety, depression, or irritability?
- ❏ Seem to be frequently tired or lack motivation?
- ❏ Sometimes lose concentration or have poor memory?
- ❏ Have slow-growing hair and nails?
- ❏ Seem to be constantly hungry?
- ❏ Frequently get indigestion?

Check the box for each "yes" answer. If you check five or more, the chances are your child isn't getting enough amino acids. Upping her intake of protein can make all the difference.

Read on to discover how to boost your child's protein intake and boost her mental and physical energy. But to understand why amino acids are so important for your child's brain, we first need to explore what the neurotransmitters they build actually do.

KEY PLAYERS IN THE ORCHESTRA OF MIND

There are hundreds of different kinds of neurotransmitters in the brain and body, but here are the main players:

- Adrenaline, noradrenaline, and dopamine make us feel good, stimulating us, motivating us, and helping us deal with stress.
- GABA counteracts these stimulating neurotransmitters by relaxing us and calming us down after stress.

- Serotonin keeps us happy, improving our mood and banishing the blues.
- Acetylcholine keeps our brain sharp, improving memory and mental alertness.
- Tryptamines keep us connected. For example, melatonin keeps us in sync with day and night and the seasons.

Many other substances in the brain act much like neurotransmitters, such as endorphins, which give us a sense of euphoria after exercise, for example. But the ones above are the big five—the key players in the orchestra. And your child's mood, memory, and mental alertness are all affected by their activity.

If serotonin is up, for example, your child is likely to be happy; if dopamine and adrenaline are down, she is likely to feel unmotivated and tired. Having the right balance of these key neurotransmitters is a must if you want your child to be in tip-top mental health, and supplementing the right amino acids can solve a wide variety of mental health problems in children.

And how do the amino acids do the job? Their action is very similar to that of prescribed drugs that directly affect neurotransmitters. For instance, amphetamines such as Ritalin work by causing an excessive release of adrenaline, whereas SSRI antidepressants like Prozac or Zoloft effectively raise levels of serotonin by preventing its breakdown in the body. But these drugs have many undesirable side effects, essentially working against our body's natural design, not with it. And SSRI antidepressants are also falling out of favor, particularly regarding use in children, as more and more studies show the benefits do not outweigh the risks, which can include suicidal thoughts and behavior.[2]

Nutrients such as amino acids work just as well, if not better, but don't have the side effects: after all, it's part of the brain and body's natural design to use them. So the best way to tune up your child's brain is to ensure she has an adequate intake of amino acids in her diet. First and foremost, this means eating enough protein every day.

POWER OF PROTEIN

The quality of a protein is determined by its balance of amino acids. Though there are twenty-three amino acids from which the body can build everything from a neurotransmitter to a muscle cell, only eight are known as essential, because they only come through diet. The other fifteen can be made in the body from the essential eight if there is not enough of them in the diet. The better the balance of amino acids—expressed as a unit known as NPU (net protein usability)—the more you can make use of the protein.

The chart opposite shows the top twenty-four individual foods and food combinations in terms of NPUs, or protein quality. Combining lentils or beans with rice, for example, is a great way of increasing the overall quality of the protein because the amino acids rice is low in, lentils and beans are rich in, and vice versa. It also shows how much of a food, or food combination, you need to eat to get a 20 g serving of protein. Your child needs to eat one or two of these servings a day, depending on her age (see below).

Protein Requirement by Age

	2–3 years	4–8 years	9–13 years	14–18 years (girls)	14–18 years (boys)
Protein (g)	13	19	34	46	52

A typical day's protein for a six-year-old might therefore include two of any of the following: an egg (10 g), a 2-ounce (50 g) serving of salmon, a 2-ounce (60 g) handful of seeds and nuts, or a 3.5-ounce (100 g) serving of beans.

For a vegetarian child, a typical day's worth might be any two of the following: a 6-ounce (170 g) container of yogurt, a handful of seeds or nuts, a 5-ounce (140 g) serving of tofu, a small cup (100 g) of quinoa, or a small serving (100 g) of beans with rice. The trick for vegetarians is to eat seed foods—that is, foods that would grow if you planted them, which includes seeds, nuts, beans, lentils, peas, corn, or the germ of grains such as wheat or oat. Flower foods, such as broccoli or cauliflower, are also relatively rich in protein.

Packed with Protein: The Top 24

Food	Percentage of calories as protein	How much for 0.75 oz (20 g)	Protein quality (NPU)
Grains/Legumes			
Quinoa	16	7 oz (200 g)/ 2 cups cooked weight	Excellent
Tofu	40	10 oz (285 g)/ 1 package	Reasonable
Corn	4	1 lb 2 oz (500 g)/ 3³/₄ cups cooked weight	Reasonable
Brown rice	5	14 oz (400 g)/ 3³/₄ cups cooked weight	Excellent
Chickpeas	22	4 oz (115 g)/ ³/₄ cup cooked weight	Reasonable
Lentils	28	3 oz (85 g)/ 1¹/₄ cups cooked weight	Reasonable
Fish/Meat			
Tuna, canned	61	3 oz (85 g)/ 1 small can	Excellent
Cod	60	1.25 oz (35 g)/ 1 very small piece	Excellent
Salmon	50	3.5 oz (100 g)/ 1 small piece	Excellent
Sardines	49	3.5 oz (100 g)/ 1 baked	Excellent
Chicken	63	2.5 oz (75 g)/ 1 small roasted breast	Excellent
Nuts/Seeds			
Sunflower seeds	15	6.5 oz (185 g)/ 1¹/₄ cups	Reasonable
Pumpkinseeds	21	2.5 oz (75 g)/ 10 tablespoons	Reasonable

(continued)

Packed with Protein, continued

Food	Percentage of calories as protein	How much for 0.75 oz (20 g)	Protein quality (NPU)
Nuts/Seeds (*continued*)			
Cashew nuts	12	4 oz (115 g)/ 1¹/₄ cups	Reasonable
Almonds	13	4 oz (115 g)/ 1¹/₄ cups	Reasonable
Eggs/Dairy			
Eggs	34	4 oz (115 g)/ 2 medium	Excellent
Yogurt, natural	22	1 lb (450 g)/ 3 small containers	Excellent
Cottage cheese	49	4.5 oz (125 g)/ 1 small container	Excellent
Vegetables			
Peas, frozen	26	9 oz (250 g)/ 2¹/₂ cups	Reasonable
Other beans	20	7 oz (200 g)/ 2¹/₂ cups	Reasonable
Broccoli	50	1.5 oz (40 g)/ ³/₄ cup	Reasonable
Spinach	49	1.5 oz (40 g)/ ³/₄ cup	Reasonable

Be aware, though, that your child can have too much protein: more doesn't always mean better. Once daily protein intake goes above 3 ounces (85 g) a day (depending on your child's current growth pattern and exercise level, hence requirement) this can have negative health consequences.

For instance, the breakdown products of protein, such as ammonia, are toxic to the body and stress the kidneys during elimination. Also, too many amino acids mean too much acid in the blood, which the body neutralizes by releasing calcium from bone. It is now well established that diets very high in protein contribute to kidney disease and osteoporosis. So, as with all else in nutrition, balance is important.

Supplementing Amino Acids

If your child is eating a reasonable amount of protein (and chewing it thoroughly), she should be getting all the amino acids that she needs. But if she is having particular problems with mood or memory, you can consider supplementation (more on this in part 3). Tests to measure levels of amino acids in the blood are available through a nutritionist (see Resources, page 217), who may then recommend supplementation of particular amino acids based on the results.

> **In summary, here are some general guidelines to help ensure your child has an optimal intake of amino acids:**
>
> - Give her between one and two servings of the protein-rich foods shown in the preceding table every day, depending on her age.
> - Include some protein with every meal, such as chickpeas or chicken in her pasta sauce or nuts and seeds with her cereal.
> - Choose good vegetable protein sources, including beans, lentils, quinoa, tofu (soy), and flower vegetables such as broccoli.
> - If your child is eating animal protein, choose free-range eggs, fish, or lean meat and go for organic whenever possible.

(continued)

Chapter 6

Why Vitamins and Minerals Make Your Child Brainy

In every great production, there are hundreds of people behind the scenes supporting the main players. The same is true of your child's brain—it's just that the heroes behind the lights, camera, and action are vitamins and minerals, rather than technicians and casting agents.

One of the main roles of vitamins and minerals is to help turn glucose into energy, amino acids into neurotransmitters, simple essential fats into more complex fats like GLA or DHA, and choline and serine into phospholipids. They are key to the task of building and rebuilding the brain and nervous system, and keeping everything running smoothly.

As we have long known, they're an essential for your child's brain. As we mentioned in the introduction, back in the early 1980s we decided to test what would happen to the intelligence of schoolchildren if given an optimal intake of vitamins and minerals. Gwillym Roberts, a headmaster and nutritional therapist from the Institute for Optimum Nutrition in London, and Professor David Benton, a psychologist from Swansea University in Wales, devised a test putting sixty schoolchildren onto a special multivitamin and mineral supplement designed to ensure an optimal intake of key nutrients.[1] Half of the children took a placebo, but the children, their parents, their teachers, and the researchers didn't know which children were taking the vitamins and minerals and which were taking the placebo.

After eight months on the supplements, the nonverbal IQs in those taking the supplements had risen by over 10 points! No changes were seen in those on the placebos. This study, published in *The Lancet* medical journal in 1988, has since been proven many times in other studies. Most have used RDA levels of nutrients, which are much lower than those in our original study, but still show increases in IQ averaging 4.5 points.

Why do vitamins and minerals raise IQ? The answer appears to be that children think faster and can concentrate for longer with an optimal intake of vitamins and minerals. Check your child out on the questionnaire below.

Intelligent Nutrient Check

Does your child:

- ❑ Eat fewer than five servings of fresh fruits and vegetables (excluding potato) every day?
- ❑ Eat less than one portion of a dark green vegetable a day?
- ❑ Eat fewer than three portions of fresh or dried tropical fruit a week?
- ❑ Eat seeds or seed oils (such as pumpkinseeds, sunflower seeds, tahini) or unroasted nuts less than three times a week?
- ❑ Typically not take a multivitamin and mineral supplement?
- ❑ Usually eat white bread, rice, or pasta instead of brown or whole-grain?
- ❑ Suffer from anxiety, depression, or irritability?
- ❑ Suffer from muscle cramps?
- ❑ Have white marks on more than two fingernails?
- ❑ Seem disconnected and find it difficult to relate or communicate?

Check the box for each "yes" answer. If you check five or more, the chances are your child isn't getting enough vitamins and minerals.

THE ULTIMATE HEAD START

The dividends of giving your child the vitamins and minerals he needs right from the start are enormous. That means during pregnancy (and, ideally, before conception), while breast-feeding, and also during the weaning process.

A sixteen-year study by the Medical Research Council in the UK shows just how critical optimum nutrition is in the early years. They fed 424 premature babies either a standard or an enriched milk formula containing extra protein, vitamins, and minerals. At eighteen months, those fed standard milk "were doing significantly less well" then the others, and at eight years old had IQs up to 14 points lower.[2]

In chapter 21, we give you details on how to keep your growing child optimally nourished through pregnancy and early infancy. But remember: It's never too late to increase brain-boosting vitamins and minerals in your child's diet, as you will see later.

NUTRIENTS FOR BRAIN VITALITY

Every one of the fifty known essential vitamins and minerals plays a major role in promoting mental health. In the chart below we list the most vital to the state of your child's brain, along with the symptoms you might see if your child is deficient, and the best food families to feed your child to ensure he gets enough.

Key Vitamins and Minerals for Brain Health

Nutrient	Symptoms of deficiency	Food source
B1	Poor concentration and attention	Whole grains, vegetables
B3	Depression, psychosis	Whole grains, vegetables
B5	Poor memory, stress	Whole grains, vegetables
B6	Irritability, poor memory, depression, stress	Whole grains, bananas
Folic acid	Anxiety, depression, psychosis	Green leafy vegetables
B12	Confusion, poor memory, psychosis	Meat, fish, dairy products, eggs
Vitamin C	Depression, psychosis	Vegetables, fresh fruit
Magnesium	Irritability, insomnia,	Green vegetables, nuts, seeds
Manganese	Dizziness, convulsions, depression	Nuts, seeds, tropical fruit
Zinc	Confusion, blank mind, depression, loss of appetite, lack of motivation and concentration	Oysters, nuts, seeds, fish

Other vitamins and minerals affect brain health indirectly: antioxidants, for instance, offer protection from pollution, while minerals keep depression, confusion, and insomnia at bay. We'll look at them all in more detail—but first, a glance at the B family of vitamins.

The B Vitamins

B vitamins are absolutely key to mental health in all of us, children and adults alike. The brain uses a large amount of them, and as they're water soluble and pass rapidly out of the body, even a short-term deficiency in any one of the eight Bs can result in a rapid shift in how your child thinks and feels. So it's best for him to get a regular intake throughout the day.

As you saw from the chart, this shouldn't be difficult: a wholesome, balanced diet is rich in the foods rich in Bs. The best sources of B1, B3, B5, and B6 are whole grains and vegetables (B6 is abundant in bananas, too); to keep folic acid topped up you'll need to provide plenty of spinach and other green leafy vegetables; and for B12 you'll need good protein, such as eggs and fish.

While the deficiency symptoms of B vitamins are well-known, we still do not know exactly why many of them occur. Each B vitamin has so many functions in the brain and nervous system that there are few hard proofs in this regard. But we do know one of the best indicators of deficiency—homocysteine levels (see sidebar).

B Deficiencies—The Homocysteine Link

How do you know if your child is getting enough B vitamins? One of the best gauges is homocysteine, a toxic protein found in the blood. If your child's blood levels of homocysteine are high, he is likely to be low in B6, B12, or folic acid because these vitamins help flush the protein out of the body. So he'll need to increase his Bs.

Because of this intimate inverse link between homocysteine and Bs, and the importance of Bs to brain health, your child's homocysteine level can be seen as a measure of his biological IQ.

As we mentioned in the introduction, researchers from Örebro University in Sweden compared school grades in ten core subjects with homocysteine levels in a group of 692 school children aged nine to fifteen. They found that higher homocysteine levels were strongly associated with lower grades.[3]

The ideal level of blood homocysteine for an adolescent or adult is below 6 µmol/l (6 micromoles/liter). For a child of ten or younger, the level should ideally lie below 5 µmol/l. See your doctor to have your child tested, and chapter 26 for details on supplementation to bring a high homocysteine level down into the ideal range.

VITAMIN B1 (THIAMINE)

Vitamin B1 helps turn glucose, the brain's main fuel, into energy—so one of the first symptoms of thiamine deficiency is mental and physical tiredness. Children who are low in this vitamin have a poor attention span and concentration.

David Benton, professor of psychology at the University of Swansea in Britain, one of the leading experts in nutrition and IQ, has found that low levels of thiamine correlate with poor cognitive function in young adults. His research results also show that thiamine supplementation was associated with reports of feeling more clearheaded, composed, and energetic and having faster reaction times, even in those whose thiamine status, according to the traditional criterion, was adequate.[4]

VITAMIN B3 (NIACIN)

Of all the nutrients connected with mental health, niacin or vitamin B3 is the most well-known. Niacin is recognized as crucial to blood glucose balance, and in the manufacture of both serotonin (the "happy" neurotransmitter) and melatonin (the sleep enhancer) from the amino acid tryptophan. Thus it is important in keeping your child on an even emotional and mental keel, in good spirits, and sleeping well at night.

VITAMIN B5 (PANTOTHENIC ACID)

Pantothenic acid or B5 is a potent memory booster. It is needed to make the memory-boosting neurotransmitter, acetylcholine. Supplementing extra B5, particularly with choline, can definitely sharpen your child's memory (see chapter 12).

VITAMINS B6, B12, AND FOLIC ACID

This trio, together with niacin, control a critical process in the body called methylation, which is vital in the formation of almost all neurotransmitters. Abnormal methylation lies behind many mental health problems, as we'll find out later in this book. A lack of B6, for example, means we don't make serotonin so efficiently, which could potentially lead to depression. B6 can help relieve stress too, while stress depletes B6. So, if your child is B6 deficient and stressed, he may be heading for depression.

Vitamin B12 is vital for a healthy nervous system. Without this crucial nutrient, neither the senses nor the brain can work properly. Even slightly low B12 levels have been linked to poor mental performance in adolescents.[5]

Getting enough B6, B12, and folic acid is absolutely vital in pregnancy too, both for protecting against developmental problems such as spina bifida and for general mental development. Children born to mothers deficient in folic acid show delayed intellectual development.[6] Since folic acid fortification of food was introduced, there has been a marked reduction in the incidence of folic acid deficiency.

As you'll have gathered, these nutrients have so many critical roles to play in the brain and nervous system that ensuring your child is getting optimal levels is really a prerequisite for mental health.

Antioxidants—Protecting Your Child's Brain

We live in a highly polluted world, and there may not be a lot you can do to avoid many of the pollutants. But you can protect your child's brain from the inside, with antioxidants.

Antioxidants are the antidote to oxidants, also known as free radicals—highly unstable molecules that can trigger cellular damage. They are a by-product of normal body processes and of combustion. In the body, oxidants are produced every time glucose is "burned" within a cell to make energy, and they can go on to damage the essential fats, proteins, and phospholipids that make up your child's brain and nervous system. Oxidants can appear in the environment, as when a car burns gasoline as fuel.

If we see oxidants as the sparks from something burning, such as food frying or a smoking cigarette, antioxidants are like fireproof gloves that prevent the sparks from damaging your brain and other tissues.

A single puff of a cigarette contains a trillion oxidants, which rapidly travel into the brain; this is why smoking around children is especially harmful. Less avoidable are the oxidants from exhaust fumes, particularly diesel. These have an insidious effect on your child's body and brain, and that is why it's crucial for your child to have a good intake of antioxidants.

Most important for the brain is the fat-based antioxidant vitamin E, which prevents the chain reactions of damage caused when oxidants enter the brain. Vitamin E is properly called d-alpha tocopherol, and its relatives gamma-tocopherol and tocotrienols are also important for the brain. These are found only in the better-quality supplements that contain vitamin E together with mixed tocopherols. They are also present in vitamin E–rich foods, such as seeds, cold-pressed seed oils, and fish.

There are other vital antioxidants. Vitamin C, for example, helps recycle vitamin E once it has grabbed hold of an oxidant. Of course, vitamin C does much more than protect your child from pollution. It has many roles to play in the brain, such as helping to balance neurotransmitters.

Among the many members of this firefighting team, the main ones are shown in figure 10, which illustrates how the body detoxifies an oxidant from fried food.

To give your child maximum protection, it's worth making sure his daily supplement contains antioxidants, as well as giving him foods high in them, such as:

- Beta-carotene—carrots, yams, dried apricots (soaked first), squash, watercress
- Vitamin C—broccoli, peppers, kiwifruit, berries, tomatoes, citrus fruit

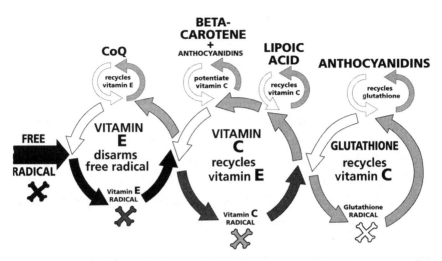

Figure 10. How antioxidants disarm an oxidant

- Vitamin E—seeds and their cold-pressed oils, wheat germ, nuts, beans, fish
- Selenium—oysters, Brazil nuts, seeds, molasses, tuna, mushrooms
- Glutathione—tuna, legumes, nuts, seeds, garlic, onions
- Anthocyanidins—berries, cherries, red grapes, beets, prunes
- Lipoic acid—red meat, potatoes, carrots, yams, beets, spinach
- Coenzyme Q—sardines, mackerel, nuts, seeds

But be aware that maximizing your child's mental powers isn't just about what your child eats. It's also about what he doesn't eat. As well as the oxidants we all make just from burning glucose as fuel, eating a piece of crispy meat introduces millions of these culprits. So it is important not to overcook, burn, or char food. A barbecue is great fun, but do cook on lower flames and ensure your child's meat is gently browned and cooked all the way through—not charred black on the outside. If you like to fry food, try sautéing it gently on low heat with the lid on the pan. If the oil spits or smokes in the frying pan, it's too hot.

Mineral Marvels

Vitamins get a lot of the good press, but certain minerals are key to brain health, helping your child calm down, grow, and get through puberty with less stress—to name just a few benefits. Let's look at them now.

CALCIUM AND MAGNESIUM

Giving your child a mineral may be the last thing you'd think of doing to calm and relax him and help him sleep. Yet that's precisely what calcium and magnesium do, by helping to relax nerve and muscle cells.

Muscle cramps are an obvious sign of magnesium deficiency. A lack of either calcium or magnesium can also make children more nervous, irritable, and aggressive. Magnesium has been used successfully to treat autistic and hyperactive children, together with other nutrients. Most of all, it helps them to sleep.

Magnesium is typically the second most commonly deficient mineral after zinc (see below) in children. Green, leafy vegetables are rich in it because it is part of the chlorophyll molecule, which gives plants their green color. So are nuts and seeds, particularly sesame, sunflower, and pumpkin. An ideal intake of magnesium is probably 500 mg a day, which is almost double what most people achieve. But it's not hard to do: 1 tablespoon of seeds a day, plus 100 mg in a multimineral, is a good way to ensure your child is getting enough.

ZINC

The most commonly deficient mineral, and one of the most critical nutrients for mental health, is zinc. This deficiency is particularly problematic and likely for children since zinc is necessary for growth. A deficiency in this mineral is associated with hyperactivity, autism, depression, anxiety, anorexia, schizophrenia, and delinquency—in short, it's implicated in a wide range of mental health problems. Astonishingly, according to the Third National Health and Nutrition Examination Survey, about half of all American children have inadequate zinc intake from their diet.[7]

Zinc has several crucial roles to play in brain development and maintenance, not least the prevention of oxidation and the synthesis of serotonin and melatonin.[8] Even healthy normal children appear to benefit from extra zinc, as demonstrated in North Dakota. Researchers gave zinc supplements to 209 seventh-grade children. They found that those taking 20 mg of zinc a day had faster, more accurate memory retrieval and better attention spans within three months than those taking 10 mg (the RDA) or a placebo.[9]

There are also many times during their development when children need a boost from extra zinc because of growth spurts, puberty, stress, infections, excess copper, blood sugar problems, and even an inherited need for more of this mineral. Boys need extra zinc from about age twelve, as zinc in their bodies is concentrated in sperm. Two sure signs of zinc deficiency are stretch marks and white spots on the fingernails, an increasingly common phenomenon seen in teenage girls and boys.

You'll find zinc in any seed food—nuts, seeds, and the germ of grains. Meat and fish are rich sources, but none is richer than oysters: a single oyster can provide as much as 15 mg of zinc!

Here are a few simple steps you can take to ensure your child gets plenty of vitamins and minerals:

- Make sure your child eats plenty of foods rich in antioxidants— fruits, vegetables, seeds, and fish. His diet should include at least five, and ideally seven, servings of fresh fruits and vegetables a day.
- Serve nuts and seeds daily, and choose whole foods, such as whole grains, lentils, beans, and brown rice, rather than refined food.
- Make sure your child takes an optimum nutrition multivitamin and mineral every day (see chapter 26 for guidance on the ideal formula depending on your child's age).
- Don't smoke, and keep your child away from smoky places, to avoid overexposure to oxidants.

Chapter 7

Don't Let Your Child Be a Heavy Metal Kid

In the last chapter we looked at some of the minerals essential to your child's mental and physical health. But not all minerals are good news. Some, such as the heavy metals lead and mercury, are thoroughly bad news if they find their way into your child's brain and nervous system. High intakes of cadmium and mercury can have a disastrous effect on intelligence and behavior in children and adults alike.

A high intake of heavy metals in children has been associated with mood swings, poor impulse control and aggressive behavior, poor attention span, depression and apathy, disturbed sleep patterns, and impaired memory and intellectual performance. If your child has symptoms like these, we recommend you have her tested for heavy metals. If these are found, you'll need to remove the source and provide the right nutrients to help detoxify your child's mind and body.

Nine-year-old Antony is a case in point. He had been diagnosed with dysgraphia—a learning difficulty that specifically affects handwriting. His parents had already noticed that his writing was directly affected by sugar and additives and had already taken these out of his diet to good effect. We conducted a hair analysis, which showed that he had high levels of the toxic metal mercury in his hair. We increased his intake of zinc, selenium, and vitamin C to help his body remove the mercury, and three months later Antony and his mother were happy to report that he'd had a significant improvement in his handwriting.

Here are some examples of heavy metals, the effect they have on mental health, where they originate, and the nutritional protectors against them.

Antinutrient	Effect	Source	Protector
Cadmium	Aggression, confusion	Cigarettes	Vitamin C, zinc
Mercury	Headaches, memory loss	Pesticides, fillings, vaccinations	Selenium
Aluminum	Associated with senility	Cookware, water	Zinc, magnesium
Copper	Anxiety and phobia	Water pipes	Zinc
Lead	Hyperactivity, aggression, low IQ	Exhaust fumes	Vitamin C, zinc

Now let's take a closer look at just what these culprits can do to our children's mental health.

HEAVY METALS—THE USUAL SUSPECTS

You might think you'd be exposed to heavy metals only if you lived or worked near a toxic dumping ground or the like. The shock is discovering how common they are in the environment.

Cadmium—Peril as You Puff

Cigarette smoke is laden with cadmium, a heavy metal associated with disturbed mental performance and increased aggression. This nasty also lurks in car exhaust fumes. There can also be small amounts in food, especially if it's refined, because beneficial minerals that act as cadmium protectors, such as selenium, are taken out during the refining process. Cadmium also knocks out zinc, so passive smokers will need more.

Keep your child away from cigarette smoke. If you smoke, quit—this is the best way to prevent your child from picking up the habit while also protecting her from heavy metal contamination.

Aluminum—Toxic Takeaway

Aluminum is found in a staggering array of modern products. Aluminum trays and foils are widely used as food packaging by supermarkets, fast-food outlets, and other food-handling operations, and the stuff also turns up in many common household products. It's in antacids, toothpaste tubes, pots and pans, even our water.

Not all aluminum will enter the body, however. Only under certain circumstances will aluminum leach from a pan, for example. Old-fashioned aluminum cookware, if used to heat something acidic like tea, tomatoes, or rhubarb, will leach particles of aluminum into the water. Also, the more zinc deficient you are, the more aluminum you absorb.

To be safe, it's best not to broil food directly on aluminum foil. Instead, use a broiling tray.

Mercury—Why Hatters Were Mad

"Mad as a hatter"—the phrase seems to have originated in the nineteenth century, when mercury compounds were used to make felt for hats. When the felt was boiled then steamed into shape, hatmakers absorbed the mercury-laden fumes. Their "madness" was caused by mercury's disturbance of brain processes, which can cause depression, irritability, loss of coordination, and other distressing symptoms.

This heavy metal is, in fact, very toxic indeed. Small amounts reach us from contaminated foods, pharmaceuticals, cosmetics, and amalgam tooth fillings. Mercury is also present in thimerosal, a preservative that was once commonly used in vaccines. Thimerosal use is being phased out by the FDA, and currently almost all vaccines that are given to children are thimerosal free.

Of particular concern is fish caught in polluted waters. All five Great Lakes and over 2,500 other North American lakes have fish consumption warnings due to mercury contamination. In March 2001, the FDA released a consumer advisory that warned pregnant women not to eat shark, swordfish, king mackerel, or tilefish, because they contain enough mercury to damage the fetus's nervous system. Young children, nursing mothers, and women who may become pregnant were advised to avoid those fish as well. Larger fish like tuna and marlin that are higher up the food chain tend to have higher levels of mercury too.

Oily fish such as tuna are a valuable source of omega-3 essential fats, however (see chapter 3). The FDA website has an up-to-date list of mercury levels found in a wide variety of fish, enabling you to choose from that list the oily fish that has the lowest levels of mercury. Check local advisories about the safety of fish caught by family and friends in your local lakes, rivers, and coastal areas.

The Copper Controversy

Copper is both an essential mineral and a toxic one. It's rare to be deficient in copper, except for people whose diets are very high in refined foods, largely because of the widespread use of copper water pipes. These leach small amounts of copper into the water. However, if you live in a soft-water area or in a house with new copper piping that hasn't yet become calcified, your family can be exposed to toxic levels of copper.

Copper and zinc are enemies. So if your child is zinc deficient, she may not be able to get rid of any excess copper.

Lead—Trouble in Mind

In the 1990s, there were a number of important studies that consistently showed lower IQ in children whose blood, hair, or baby teeth contained the highest levels of lead. When Herbert Needleman, an associate professor of child psychiatry, conducted a follow-up study of children who'd had elevated lead levels eleven years earlier, he found a sevenfold increase in the odds of failure to graduate from high school, lower class standing, greater absenteeism, more reading disabilities, and poor vocabulary, fine motor skills, reaction time, and hand-eye coordination.[1]

Fortunately, since the advent of unleaded gasoline, lead is much less of a problem these days. Some lead remains in the environment, but the most likely source these days is drinking water from old lead pipes. Symptoms of lead toxicity include lowered IQ, aggression, and headaches.

HOW TO HANDLE THE HEAVIES

We've seen the problem. Now, how to fix it? First you need to discover which, if any, toxic minerals are affecting your child.

Hair Mineral Analysis: The Heavy Metal Tune-Up

There's a simple way to find out if these heavy and toxic minerals are affecting your child—a hair mineral analysis. By analyzing a small amount of hair, your child can be effectively screened not only for the bad guys, such as lead, cadmium, mercury, and aluminum, but also for the good guys, such as magnesium, zinc, chromium, manganese, and so on. Screening can be arranged through your naturopath or nutritionist.

But what do you do if your child has raised levels of toxic minerals? Luckily, many essential minerals have an antagonistic relationship with heavy metals, meaning that taking more of the essential minerals depletes the toxic ones. So once you've done a hair analysis, it's worth getting tailored advice on how to detox your child. See Resources on page 217 for details on how to locate a suitable naturopath or nutritionist near you.

Foods That Fight Heavy Metals

Meanwhile, you can certainly improve your child's detoxification, if she needs it, by following the general nutrition guidelines in this book and ensuring she gets plenty of antioxidants from fresh fruits and vegetables and plenty of water.

In terms of specific foods, there are a few that can help keep your child's brain "clean." Garlic, onions, and eggs include sulfur-containing amino acids, specifically methionine and cystine, which protect against mercury, cadmium, and lead toxicity. Pectin in apples, carrots, and citrus fruits also helps to remove heavy metals—yet another reason for an apple a day!

In summary, here are some general guidelines to help keep your child free from heavy metals:

- Supplement with a multivitamin and mineral including zinc, selenium, and vitamin C for toxic mineral protection—see chapter 26 for our specific supplement recommendations.
- Have a mineral analysis of your child's hair, available through naturopaths or nutritionists (see Resources).

Chapter 8

Keeping Your Child Chemical Free

About 3,000 food additives have been approved by the FDA. That's 150 to 160 pounds of additives consumed by an average American every year![1] In addition, gallons of pesticides and herbicides are sprayed on and around fruits and vegetables, and thousands of chemicals are introduced into our homes. Some of our children, indeed perhaps all of us, aren't coping well with this chemical onslaught.

All these compounds are classified as antinutrients—substances that interfere with our ability to either absorb or use essential nutrients, or in some cases, that promote the loss of essential nutrients from the body.

A high intake of antinutrient chemicals has been associated with mood swings, poor impulse control and aggressive behavior, poor attention span, depression and apathy, disturbed sleep patterns, and impaired memory and intellectual performance. The best way to remedy or indeed prevent these kinds of symptoms is to keep these chemicals out of your child's diet as much as possible.

BATTLING THE ADDITIVE BLUES

Let's take a look at tartrazine, which is still added into many popular soft drinks for children to color them yellow or orange, yet it has been consistently linked to hyperactivity in children. And, in fact, a closer look at this food chemical reveals something rather sinister.

Dr. Neil Ward from the University of Surrey in the UK decided to test what happens to minerals when drinks containing tartrazine were consumed.

He gave children drinks that looked and tasted identical, some with tartrazine and some without. He found that adding tartrazine to drinks increased the amount of zinc excreted in the urine, perhaps by binding to zinc in the blood and preventing it from being used by the body.[2]

In this study, like many others, he also found emotional and behavioral changes in every child who consumed tartrazine. Four out of the ten children in the study had severe reactions, three experiencing an outbreak of eczema or having an asthma attack within forty-five minutes of ingestion. Tartrazine is one of the first of over 1,000 chemical food additives proven to be an antinutrient.

Researchers at the University of Southampton in the UK investigated the effect of artificial food colorings and a preservative in the diet of 1,873 three-year-old children. They found that the children's behavior was worse when the food colorings (a mixture of sunset yellow, tartrazine, carmoisine, and ponceau 4R) and preservative (sodium benzoate) were in their diet than not. Interestingly, the effect was no different for children who had previously been identified as hyperactive compared with those who were not.[3] The same additives and preservative were tested again, this time with the addition of the color Allura red, in an almost identical study to confirm the findings. The results were strikingly similar, with signs of hyperactivity seen in all 153 three-year-old and 144 eight- and nine-year-old children who were not hyperactive at the outset.[4]

The primary reasons for adding chemicals to food is to make the food look better by changing its color and to preserve and stabilize it. Most of the additives are synthetic compounds, some with known negative health effects. But more important, we don't know what the long-term consequences of consuming such large amounts of additives are; this is especially true for children, whose brains and bodies are still developing. It is therefore best to avoid all additives, with a few notable exceptions. These are:

- Colors: vitamin B2 (riboflavin), carotene
- Antioxidants: vitamin C (ascorbic acid), vitamin E (tocopherols)
- Emulsifier: lecithin
- Stabilizers: vitamin B3 (niacin), pectin

The chart below gives the most up-to-date information on the worst of the food additives. In many cases, it's not possible to say with any certainty how these foods might affect your child's mental health.

However, since the brain is not separate from the body, we know that any substance that can have such a negative effect on physical health is likely to having a negative effect on mental and emotional health. There is a distinct lack of research in this area because food manufacturers have no desire to carry out studies beyond the minimum requirements to enable them to put these additives into food.

Top 20 Additives to Avoid

Allura red AC

How used: Widely used as food coloring, in sodas, snacks, sauces, preserves, soups, wine, cider, and so forth.

What you need to know: Avoid if your child has asthma, rhinitis (including hay fever), or urticaria (an allergic rash also known as hives). Banned in some European countries.

Aspartame

How used: Widely used as a sweetener in snacks, candy, desserts, diet foods.

What you need to know: Aspartame may affect people with PKU (phenylketonuria). Recent reports show the possibility of headaches, blindness, and seizures with long-term, high-dose aspartame.

Benzoic acid

How used: Widely used preservative in many foods, including drinks, low-sugar products, cereals, meat products.

What you need to know: Can temporarily inhibit the function of digestive enzymes and may deplete glycine levels. Should be avoided by those with allergic conditions such as hay fever, hives, or asthma.

Butylated hydroxyanisole (BHA)

How used: Very widely used as a preservative, particularly in fat-containing foods, confectionery, meats.

What you need to know: The International Agency for Research on Cancer says that BHA is possibly carcinogenic to humans. BHA also interacts with nitrites to form chemicals known to be mutagenic (that is, that cause changes in the DNA of cells).

Calcium benzoate

How used: Preservative in many foods, including drinks, low-sugar products, cereals, meat products.

What you need to know: Can temporarily inhibit the function of digestive enzymes and may deplete levels of the amino acid glycine. Should be avoided by those with hay fever, hives, or asthma.

Calcium sulfite

How used: Mainly as a preservative in a vast array of foods from burgers to cookies.

What you need to know: Sulfites can cause bronchial problems, flushing or reddening of the skin, low blood pressure, tingling, and anaphylactic shock. The International Labour Organization (ILO) says to avoid them if you suffer from bronchial asthma, cardiovascular or respiratory problems, or emphysema.

Monosodium glutamate (MSG)

How used: Widely used as a flavor enhancer.

What you need to know: Those sensitive to monosodium glutamate have felt symptoms including pressure on the head, seizures, chest pains, headache, nausea, burning sensations, and tightness of face.

Potassium benzoate

How used: See calcium benzoate (above).

What you need to know: See calcium benzoate (above).

Potassium nitrate

How used: Used as a preservative in cured meats and canned meat products.

What you need to know: Three main health concerns: it can lower the oxygen-carrying capacity of the blood; it may combine with other substances to form nitrosamines, which are carcinogenic; and it may have an atrophying effect on the adrenal gland.

Propyl p-hydroxybenzoate, propylparaben, paraben

How used: Preservatives in cereals, snacks, paté, meat products, and confectionery.

What you need to know: Parabens have been identified as the cause of chronic dermatitis in numerous instances.

Saccharin and its sodium, potassium, and calcium salts

How used: Very widely used sweetener, found in diet and no-added-sugar products.

What you need to know: The International Agency for Research on Cancer has concluded that saccharin is possibly carcinogenic to humans.

Sodium metabisulfite

How used: Widely used as a preservative and antioxidant.

What you need to know: May provoke life-threatening asthma.

Sodium sulfite

How used: Preservative used in wine making and processed foods.

What you need to know: Sulfites have been associated with triggering asthma attacks. Most asthmatics are sensitive to sulfites in food.

Stannous chloride (tin)

How used: Antioxidant and color-retention agent in canned and bottled foods, fruit juices.

What you need to know: Acute poisoning has been reported from ingestion of fruit juices containing concentrations of tin greater than 250 mg/l, causing nausea, vomiting, diarrhea, and headaches.

Sulfur dioxide

How used: Very widely used preservative.

What you need to know: Sulfur dioxide reacts with a wide range of substances found in food, including various vitamins, minerals, enzymes, and essential fats. The most common adverse reaction to sulfites is bronchial problems, particularly in those prone to asthma. Other adverse reactions may include hypotension (low blood pressure), flushing, tingling sensations, and anaphylactic shock. The ILO says you should avoid sulfur dioxide if you suffer from conjunctivitis, bronchitis, emphysema, bronchial asthma, or cardiovascular disease.

Sunset yellow FCF, orange yellow S

How used: Widely used food coloring.

What you need to know: Some animal studies have indicated growth retardation and severe weight loss. People with asthma, rhinitis, or urticaria should avoid this product.

Tartrazine

How used: Widely used yellow food color.

What you need to know: May cause allergic reactions in perhaps 15 percent of the population. It may be a cause of asthmatic attacks and has been implicated in bouts of hyperactivity disorder in children. Those who suffer from asthma, rhinitis, and urticaria may find symptoms worsen after consumption.

Source: P. Cox and P. Brusseau, *Secret Ingredients* (Bantam, 1997), with permission of Peter Cox and Bantam Books.

See chapter 23 for more details of what to look for on labels.

GO FOR ORGANIC

The presence of pesticide residue, particularly on fruits and vegetables, is a widely acknowledged fact. Again, it's difficult to say how significant the impact on your child's health might be. But since any toxic substance will affect all parts of the body, including the brain to some extent, it seems wise to try to avoid pesticides as much as possible.

The best way to do this is to give organic produce to your child whenever you can. And of course, organic food also contains higher amounts of health-giving nutrients. Some organic food is much more expensive than conventionally grown food, but in some cases there is little difference in price, so do what you can within your budget. Most organic food hasn't been forced to grow fast and consequently has less water and more dry weight in it. So three organic carrots would fill you up as much as four regular supermarket carrots.

It's value for money: even if the price is 25 percent more, you're getting just as much carrot at the end of the day, plus all the extra nutrients and no pesticide or herbicide residues.

But is it better to eat organic apples flown all the way from South America or conventionally grown American apples that have not traveled so far? Quite a conundrum! By buying fruits and vegetables that are in season, you are more likely to be able to get food that is both local and organic. That means apples and pears in winter, and blackberries and plums in summer, for example. Also, go for whole lettuces rather than bagged lettuces since these are less likely to be chemically treated to maintain freshness.

Organic means much more than pesticide free. Those who raise organic meat, poultry, or fish have to adhere to strict rules, not only about the feed but also about how animals are reared and the use of any growth hormones or antibiotics. It's well worth paying the extra for organic meat, eggs, farmed fish, or milk.

To help prevent your child from being exposed to additives, do the following:

- Avoid foods containing chemical food additives.
- Be vigilant when buying food and drink.
- Stick to whole, natural foods as much as possible, since these should be additive free. You will still need to check the label.
- Choose organic food, including meat, eggs, milk, fish, fruit, and vegetables.

Chapter 9

Protecting Your Child from Brain Allergies

As many as one in five adults and children, and probably one in three with behavioral problems, are sensitive or have allergic reactions to common foods such as milk, wheat, yeast, and eggs.[1] Yet the knowledge that allergy to foods and chemicals can adversely affect moods and behavior in children has been widespread, but ignored, for a very long time.

Back in the 1980s, researchers found that allergies can affect any system of the body, including the central nervous system—a result confirmed by recent double-blind controlled trials. Allergies can cause a diverse range of symptoms, from fatigue, slowed thought processes, irritability, and agitation, to aggressive behavior, nervousness, anxiety, depression, ADHD, autism, hyperactivity, and learning disabilities.[2]

> Five-year-old Veronica is a case in point. She had been diagnosed with mild autism and had also been suffering her entire life with chronic constipation and regular tummy aches. When her parents brought her to us at the Brain Bio Centre, we arranged an IgG food allergy test that revealed an allergy to gluten. When this was removed from her diet, her parents were pleased to report a major improvement in her sociability and much improved digestion with regular bowel movements and no tummy aches.

In susceptible children, these types of symptoms can be caused by a variety of substances, though many have reactions to common foods or food additives, or both. Some children, particularly those with hyperactivity or ADHD, may also react to salicylates, a natural component in many otherwise wholesome foods. This phenomenon will be covered in more detail in chapter 16.

The most convincing evidence for the wide-ranging effects of food allergies comes from a well-conducted double-blind, placebo-controlled crossover trial by Dr. Joseph Egger and his team, who studied seventy-six hyperactive children to find out whether diet can contribute to behavioral disorders. The results showed that 79 percent of the children tested reacted adversely to artificial food colorings and preservatives, primarily tartrazine and benzoic acid, which produced a marked deterioration in behavior.

However, Eggers found that no child reacted to these alone. In fact, forty-eight different foods were found to produce symptoms among the children tested. For example, 64 percent reacted to cow's milk, 59 percent to chocolate, 49 percent to wheat, 45 percent to oranges, 39 percent to eggs, 32 percent to peanuts, and 16 percent to sugar. Interestingly, it was not only the children's behavior that improved after their diets were modified; most of the associated symptoms also lessened considerably, including headaches, fits, abdominal discomfort, chronic rhinitis, aching limbs, skin rashes, and mouth ulcers.[3] Other studies have reported very similar results.[4]

These studies are prime examples of how problems created by allergies often produce a multitude of physical and mental symptoms and affect many body systems. Furthermore, allergies are very specific to the individual, as are the symptoms they create.

ALLERGY, INTOLERANCE, OR SENSITIVITY?

These days, people use the terms food allergies, food intolerances, and food sensitivities almost interchangeably. So what is the difference?

The classic definition of an allergy is simply an exaggerated physical reaction to a substance where the immune system is clearly involved. The immune system, which is the body's defense system, has the ability to produce markers for substances it doesn't like, the classic example being an antibody called IgE (immunoglobulin type E). When food containing the allergen is digested, it enters the bloodstream and meets its IgE marker, triggering the release of chemicals. These include histamine, which causes the classic symptoms of allergy—skin rashes, hay fever, rhinitis, sinusitis, asthma, eczema, and anaphylaxis (a reaction where throat and mouth swell and severe asthma comes on, sometimes accompanied by a rash, rapid dropping of blood pressure, an irregular heartbeat, and loss of consciousness).

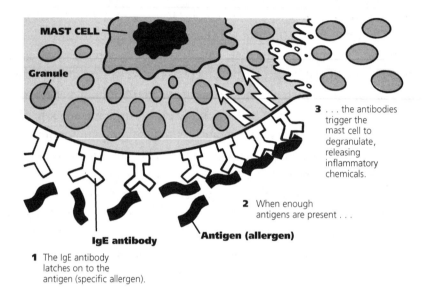

MAST CELL

Granule

3 . . . the antibodies trigger the mast cell to degranulate, releasing inflammatory chemicals.

2 When enough antigens are present . . .

IgE antibody   **Antigen (allergen)**

1 The IgE antibody latches on to the antigen (specific allergen).

Figure 11. How IgE antibodies cause allergic reactions

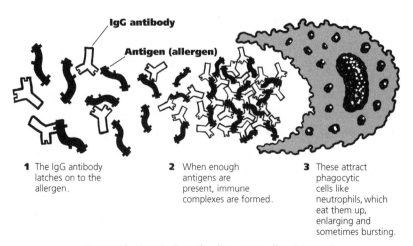

IgG antibody

Antigen (allergen)

1 The IgG antibody latches on to the allergen.

2 When enough antigens are present, immune complexes are formed.

3 These attract phagocytic cells like neutrophils, which eat them up, enlarging and sometimes bursting.

Figure 12. How IgG antibodies cause allergic reactions

All of these IgE-mediated reactions are immediate and severe and may be life threatening. If your child has this type of allergy, you probably already know about it and are keeping your child well away from the offending food.

The most common type of food allergy, however, involves a different marker—IgG. IgG allergies are often called delayed-onset, because the reactions may take anywhere from an hour to three days to show themselves. They are also usually far less dramatic, so they may just manifest as an uncomfortable feeling with no obvious cause. Add to this the fact that IgG reactions are often to widely consumed foods, and your child may well end up eating foods she's allergic to on a regular basis.

Food intolerances and sensitivities are reactions to food where there is no measurable antibody response. Examples of these include lactose intolerance, where a child lacks the enzyme to digest milk sugar, or lactose, and can develop diarrhea and abdominal discomfort from drinking milk, or intolerance to the flavor enhancer MSG, which makes some kids hyperactive.

THE TOP TEN ALLERGENS

Any food can cause an allergic reaction, but the most common include wheat and other gluten grains, milk, eggs, yeast, shellfish, nuts, peanuts, garlic, and soy. Most food allergies are a reaction to the protein in a particular food—particularly the foods we eat most frequently.

Wheat is most likely at the top of this list because it contains a substance called gliadin, which irritates the gut wall. Gliadin is a type of gluten, a sticky protein that allows pockets of air to form when combined with yeast, hence allowing bread dough to rise. Eating a lot of wheat products isn't good for anyone, and especially not for your child if she has developed an allergy. The connections between wheat allergy, autism, and ADHD are well established (see chapters 16 and 17).

Rye, barley, and oats contain much less gluten as well as different kinds of it. So if your child is allergic to wheat, she may be able to tolerate rye, barley, and oats, while some children who are allergic to wheat, rye, and barley can tolerate oats, which contains no gliadin.

Dairy products, including cheese and yogurt, cause allergic reactions in many children. Some children can seemingly tolerate goat's or sheep's milk but not cow's milk. However, this is more likely due to consuming less dairy overall: goat's and sheep's milk and cheese tend to be sold in much smaller amounts and are not universally available, after all. Allergic reactions often include a blocked nose, frequent colds, bloating and indigestion, "thick" head, fatigue, earaches, and headaches.

COMING TO GRIPS WITH ALLERGIES

Of all the avenues so far researched, the link between behavioral problems and allergy is the best established. If your child is hyperactive or prone to unexplained mood swings, allergy testing is likely to be worthwhile. Let's take a look at the options.

Allergy Tests

If your child has a history of infantile colic, eczema, asthma, ear infections, hay fever, seasonal allergies, digestive problems (including bloating, constipation, and diarrhea), frequent colds, or any behavioral or learning problems, you should suspect a delayed food allergy and should have her tested to identify the culprit. The best test is IgG ELISA, which uses a finger-prick blood sample and a home test.

Testing is best done under the guidance of a nutritionally oriented or naturopathic doctor or allergy expert, who can devise a diet for your child that cuts out all allergy-provoking foods and includes suitable alternatives. See Resources, page 217 and 218, for details on arranging allergy testing and finding a nutritionist in your area.

An alternative method of identifying food allergies is an elimination and challenge diet, which involves removing any likely culprits from your child's diet for a period of time (often from two weeks to three months) and noting any changes in behavior and mental and physical symptoms. Then the foods can be reintroduced in a controlled way while simultaneously monitoring your child's state of health. It has to be said, however, that this method has many shortcomings because the range of foods a child can react to is so broad.

As you'll already know if you or your child has an IgE allergy, the food in question (such as peanuts or shrimp) will have to be avoided for life. But IgG allergies—which have a relatively gentle, delayed effect—may not be long-term. By identifying the foods that your child is allergic to, strictly avoiding them for around six months and improving digestive health, your child may lose her allergy to them. But in some cases, an IgG allergy reaction is, like IgE allergies, for life. (If you'd like to find out more, read *Hidden Food Allergies*, by Patrick Holford and James Braly, MD.)

The Gut Factor

Digestive problems are often the underlying factor in a delayed-onset, or IgG, food allergy. Many children have excessively leaky digestive tracts, meaning that partially undigested proteins enter their bloodstream and trigger a reaction.

The leakiness can develop with frequent use of antibiotics or aspirin, gastrointestinal infection, an imbalance in gut flora, or a deficiency in essential fats, vitamin A, or zinc. So identifying and avoiding what your child is reacting to is just half the equation with an IgG food allergy. The other half is getting her digestion back into gear (see Gut Feelings, page 148, for more on this).

Children who have food allergy symptoms such as frequent ear or chest infections are likely to be prescribed antibiotics by their doctors. But antibiotics can make the gut leakier and worsen the allergy, leading in turn to more antibiotics in a vicious cycle of unnecessary ill health. Clearly, it's best to deal with the root cause of the symptoms by identifying food allergens and removing them from your child's diet rather than relying on antibiotics for short-term relief and long-term worsening of the problem.

There are a number of ways to test for, and reduce, your child's allergic potential:

- Take wheat and dairy products out of her diet strictly for one month or more and see how she feels. In any case, try to limit these food groups in your child's diet by not serving them every day.

- Improve your child's digestion by including plenty of fresh fruit, vegetables, seeds, and fish in her diet, foods that contain essential fats and zinc.
- Keep antibiotics to a minimum—they damage the digestive tract.
- If you suspect your child has a food allergy, have an IgG ELISA food allergy test and see a clinical nutritional therapist, who can test what your child is allergic to, devise a course of action to reduce her allergic potential, and ensure that your child's diet remains balanced and healthful while excluding these problem foods.

PART 2

Give Your Child a Head Start

We've talked about the various components of food that are most important in your child's diet and those to avoid. And we've shown that eating the best foods has been proven to boost IQ, improve mood and behavior, hone memory and concentration, and sharpen reading and writing skills. In this part of the book, you'll discover how to maximize your child's potential for better school performance while helping him to enjoy life and feel personally fulfilled.

Chapter 10

Testing, Testing

Are your child's mind and memory sharp? Can he concentrate and stay alert for an hour? Is his mood stable? Does he sleep well, get to sleep easily, and wake up fizzing with energy and raring to go? Or is he often exhausted, easily distracted, and prone to overreact or get upset or angry easily?

Now that you've learned the basics about the nutrients your child needs for optimum nutrition, it's time to get a handle on what your child's intelligence is all about.

First, we're all different due to our genes, and your child will inherit his own unique strengths and weaknesses. But genes are less important than you might think—they are only part of the story when it comes to how your child develops. These bits of DNA are really just the instructions inside each cell to build proteins out of the amino acids that you eat. So we inherit slightly different abilities to build certain proteins, and that in turn changes not only how we look, but also how we think. That's because proteins make enzymes and enzymes make the neurotransmitters that are so key to how we think and feel. Since proteins, enzymes, and neurotransmitters are all made from nutrients, it's no surprise to find that food directly affects the brain.

THE FACETS OF INTELLIGENCE

As we discussed in chapter 3, there are three kinds of intelligence: intellectual, emotional, and physical.

Intellectual intelligence we are well aware of. It concerns your child's ability to learn, remember, solve problems, think laterally, concentrate, and so on.

Emotional intelligence we can define as the ability to monitor one's own and others' emotions and react appropriately, channel our emotions to serve a goal, respond with empathy, and maintain healthy relationships. Being sensitive to how another child feels and saying a kind word, not overreacting when things aren't going his own way, or being able to say how he feels are all part of your child's emotional intelligence.

Physical intelligence involves overall physical fitness, balance, agility and coordination, anticipation, reaction time, strength, and flexibility. Not bumping into things and hurting yourself on a daily basis and being able to learn a physical skill are examples of physical intelligence.

All these kinds of intelligence involve the brain, yet psychological and social theories of intelligence and behavior often seem to glance over this fundamental fact. Put simply, if your child's brain isn't working properly, he can't think or feel straight. Most of the problems we humans create in our own and the larger world come about when we don't think clearly, and then respond with inappropriate emotional reactions. To look at it another way, whatever your archetype of an enlightened person might be—whether Buddha or Christ, Gandhi or the Dalai Lama, Einstein or Edison—the chances are that you define their enlightenment as clear thinking and calm responding, not at the mercy of every passing emotion.

But are such qualities something we are born with, or are they acquired? And do they depend in any way on nutrition? Even though there's obviously an inherited aspect to intelligence, we are going to show you how optimum nutrition promotes all-around intelligence by nourishing your child's brain.

Before doing so, here's a simple checklist of questions to help you gauge your child's current mental, emotional, and physical state. Given that age is going to determine ability, please answer these questions, where appropriate, in relation to other children's ability at the same age, or to your child's school peers.

YOUR CHILD'S BRAIN CHECK

Concentration and focus

- ❏ Is your child often restless and overactive?
- ❏ Does your child disturb other people?
- ❏ Does your child fail to finish things he starts?
- ❏ Does your child constantly fidget or squirm when he's meant to be still?
- ❏ Is your child inattentive or easily disturbed?
- ❏ Does your child get dizzy or irritable if he doesn't eat often?

IQ, memory, and creative thinking

- ❏ Would you describe your child as a slow learner?
- ❏ Does he lose the plot in films or stories?
- ❏ Does he find it hard to do calculations in his head (age six plus)?
- ❏ Does he find it hard to make up imaginary stories?
- ❏ Would you describe your child as forgetful?
- ❏ Is your child able to entertain himself if left alone?

Reading and writing

- ❏ Is your child behind in school with his reading?
- ❏ Is your child behind in school in his writing?
- ❏ If you ask him, does your child say that the words move on the page?
- ❏ Is his spelling particularly bad or does he get the letters in the wrong place?
- ❏ Does he frequently get left and right confused?
- ❏ Has your child been suspected or confirmed as dyslexic?

Mood and behavior

- ❏ Is your child especially excitable and impulsive?
- ❏ Does he expect his demands to be immediately met?
- ❏ Does he become easily frustrated?

❏ Is he prone to outbursts of temper or acting out?

❏ Does your child's mood change quickly and is he often unhappy?

❏ Does your child cry easily and often?

Physical coordination

❏ Would you describe your child as clumsy?

❏ Does your child frequently have cuts and bruises and bump into things?

❏ Is he incompetent with ball sports?

❏ Is he slow to learn physical activities?

❏ Can he throw a ball 3 feet in the air, clap, and catch it (age six plus)?

❏ Does he have difficulty with activities that involve balance?

Check the box for each "yes" answer. If you check three or more "yes" answers in any of these sections, or have a total score over 10 (the maximum score is 25), then it's very likely that following our recommendations will help your child think and feel better.

The following four chapters explain what steps you can take to optimize your child's potential.

Chapter 11

Thinking Faster, Boosting IQ

It may surprise you to know that you can boost your child's intelligence quotient or IQ score at any age. Some people argue that your real intelligence—how smart you are—is innate, something you're born with. But the truth is that your ability to make intelligent decisions depends not only on this aspect of intelligence but also on the clarity of your mind, how quickly you can think, your attention, how long you can concentrate, and how good your memory is. All of these can be improved with optimum nutrition.

> Twelve-year-old Rachel is a case in point. She had been diagnosed with global developmental delay at four years of age, and before coming to us at the Brain Bio Centre, her IQ was measured as 45. We assessed her nutrient status and found that she was low in many key brain nutrients, including zinc, magnesium, and the B vitamins. Her diet simply did not contain the nutrients that she needed. Improvements in her diet, such as increasing the amount of freshly prepared food that she ate and taking a high-dose multivitamin and mineral formula along with some fish oils, resulted in a 25-point increase in her IQ after ten months.

This result should not be surprising. In part 1 of this book, we saw how the brain, composed of a highly complex network of neurons, is made from what we eat. Thinking is a pattern of activity across this network. The messengers relaying the thoughts are neurotransmitters, which again are made from and directly affected by what we eat. When we learn, we actually change the wiring of the brain. When we think, we change the activity of neurotransmitters.

So we and our children shape the way we think, to a large degree; this was the logic that made us investigate, in 1986, whether giving a child an optimal intake of nutrients used by the brain and nervous system would improve intellectual performance.

FEEDING THE INTELLECT

Intellectual performance is generally measured as IQ, with a score of 100 considered to be average, no matter the age of the child being tested. About 5 percent of children score above 125, and less than 10 percent score below 80, which is considered to be educationally subnormal and in need of special help.

Way back in 1960, there was evidence of a link between IQ and nutrition. A study by Dr. Albert Kubala and colleagues in the United States showed that higher levels of vitamin C were associated with an increased IQ. Kubala divided 351 students into high– and low–vitamin C groups, depending on levels of the vitamin in their blood. The students' IQs were then measured and found to average 113 and 109 respectively: those with higher blood levels of the vitamin had IQs averaging 4.5 points higher.[1]

Then, in 1981, another researcher looked at the effect of multivitamins on children with mental disabilities. Having heard that some children with Down Syndrome had made big increases in IQ by taking multivitamins, Dr. Ruth Harrell ran the first ever double-blind trial, giving twenty-two mentally disabled children high-strength multivitamin and mineral supplements, or placebos.[2] After four months, the IQs of the children taking the supplements had improved by 5 to 10 points, while those on the placebo had shown no change. All the children were then put on the supplements, and after an additional four months, the average IQ improvement was 10.2 points.

But up to then, no one had tested the effects of vitamins on normal children in school. So in 1986 we decided to see whether giving a high-potency multivitamin would improve the IQ of ordinary British schoolchildren.

Working with Gwillym Roberts, a headmaster and nutritional therapist who had trained at the Institute for Optimum Nutrition, we worked out what combination of nutrients would optimally nourish the brain. Roberts then gave these to a pilot group of students at his school, measuring their IQs before and after. Their nonverbal IQ went up by a staggering 10 points. (Nonverbal IQ, which involves activities such as shape pattern matching, is considered more innate than verbal IQ, which varies more according to the subject's schooling and grasp of English.)

To test this further, Roberts devised a randomized, double-blind, placebo-controlled trial with David Benton, professor of psychology at Swansea University in the UK. Once again, after eight months on the supplements, the nonverbal IQs in those taking the supplements had risen by an average of over 10 points.[3]

This now famous IQ study, published in *The Lancet* medical journal, spawned more than a dozen similar studies to test the idea further. The next big one, conducted by professors Stephen Schoenthaler and John Yudkin, world-famous psychologist Hans Eysenck, and Dr. Linus Pauling, involved 615 children given much lower levels of nutrients, at RDA levels. Once again, the results showed that the simple addition of a vitamin and mineral supplement could increase IQ scores by as much as 20 points, with an average increase of at least 4.5 points, this time over three months.[4]

The truth is that a 4.5 point IQ shift would get many thousands of educationally subnormal children reclassified and returned to mainstream education. More comprehensive nutritional programs have brought even children with IQs in the 40s back into the normal range. But your child doesn't have to be in this category to benefit. Children with high IQs have also shown improvement.

The results of our earlier trials have been replicated more than a dozen times and shown to work in ten out of thirteen well-designed trials.[5] (A study at Kings College, London, which at one month was too short, showed no effect.[6]) You do, however, need to be suboptimally nourished. In other words, once you're getting your ideal intake of nutrients, more won't make you even brighter.

The consistent, positive benefit of giving your child supplements is also likely to last for life, according to a recent survey carried out by Aberdeen University's Department of Mental Health in Scotland, which found that supplement use also correlates with higher IQ scores later in life. This survey also emphasized the link between getting enough omega-3 fats and sharp intelligence.[7]

How Nutrients Boost IQ

But how exactly do nutrients increase IQ scores? Wendy Snowden, a British researcher at Reading University's psychology department, decided to investigate. Once again, schoolchildren were given supplements or a placebo.[8] After ten weeks, the children taking supplements showed significant increases in nonverbal IQ scores, but not in verbal IQ scores. A close analysis of performance in the IQ tests showed the same error rate, but the children were able to work faster and attempt more questions after the ten weeks of supplementation. For the verbal IQ test, all children completed all questions, so there was no room for improvement in work rate.

All this suggests that vitamin and mineral supplements effectively increase the speed of information processing in the brain—clearly a significant factor in IQ and, by implication, in intelligence. These amazing nutrients seem to help children think faster and also concentrate longer—which we'll explore in more detail in the next chapter.

GO-FASTER FOOD

Certain vitamins, minerals, and fats seem particularly good at boosting brain speed. Let's look at them now.

Brain-Accelerating Vitamins and Minerals

When it comes to fast cognition, there is good reason to "think zinc." A recent trial involving 209 seventh-graders in North Dakota showed remarkable results in how zinc supplements help speed up thinking.[9] The children were given a juice drink containing either 10 mg of zinc, 20 mg of zinc, or none. The RDA for zinc for this age group is 10 mg, so it's likely that these children would have been getting something like this level of the mineral.

At the beginning and end of the study, students had to perform a number of tests designed to measure mental skills, like attention, memory, problem solving, and hand-to-eye coordination.

Examples include tapping a key on the keyboard as fast as possible, using a mouse to follow an object moving across the screen, searching a group of objects for two of a kind, learning and remembering lists of words or simple geometric patterns, and categorizing objects.

Compared to the students who received no additional zinc, students given 20 mg zinc each day decreased reaction time on a visual memory test by 12 percent, versus 6 percent; increased correct answers on a word recognition test by 9 percent, versus 3 percent; and increased scores on a test requiring sustained attention and vigilance by 6 percent, versus 1 percent.

These results illustrate why the RDA level of nutrients, which is the amount needed to prevent your child from developing a deficiency disease (such as scurvy, from a lack of vitamin C), is hopelessly inadequate if you want to keep your child's brain optimally nourished. Other nutrients that boost IQ when taken beyond RDA levels include vitamins B1, B6, and B12 and folic acid. Studies with teenagers, for example, have found that 50 mg of vitamin B1 a day improves speed of thinking—yet the RDA is a mere 1 mg![10]

So how much is enough? The RDA issue points to the need to know how much of the important vitamins and minerals your child needs to take to accelerate his thinking. Some die-hard dieticians still believe the mantra that your child can get all the nutrients he needs from a well-balanced diet. While we encourage you wholeheartedly to feed your child a well-balanced diet, as defined in part 1, the evidence in dozens of studies reported in this book shows that achieving more than the basic RDA levels of nutrients will boost intelligence. And in our original study in the mid-1980s, where children were given the highest levels of vitamins and minerals, produced the biggest increase in IQ scores.

The following chart shows the levels of vitamins and minerals that we recommend you give your child every day, assuming you also ensure his diet is the best possible too.

The Ideal Daily Supplement Program

Nutrient	Unit	Age in Years						
		Less than 1	1–2	3–4	5–6	7–8	9–11	12–13
Essential Vitamins								
A (retinol)*	mcg	500	650	800	1,000	1,500	2,000	2,500
D*	mcg	3	4	5	7	9	11	12
E*	mg	13	16	20	23	30	40	50
C	mg	100	150	300	400	500	600	700
B1 (thiamine)	mg	5	6	8	12	16	20	24
B2 (riboflavin)	mg	5	6	8	12	16	20	24
B3 (niacin)	mg	7	12	16	18	20	22	24
B5 (pantothenic acid)	mg	10	15	20	25	30	35	40
B6 (pyridoxine)	mg	5	7	10	12	16	20	25
B12	mcg	5	6.5	8	9	10	10	10
Folic Acid	mcg	100	120	140	160	180	200	220
Biotin	mcg	30	45	60	70	80	90	100
Essential Minerals								
Calcium	mg	150	165	180	190	200	210	220
Magnesium	mg	50	65	80	90	100	110	120
Iron	mg	4	5.5	7	8	9	10	10
Zinc	mg	4	5.5	7	8	9	10	10
Manganese	mcg	300	350	400	500	700	1,000	1,000
Iodine	mcg	40	50	60	70	80	90	100
Chromium	mcg	15	19	23	25	27	30	30
Selenium	mcg	10	18	20	24	26	28	30
Copper	mcg	400	550	700	800	900	1,000	1,000

* To calculate IU values, please see conversions on page viii.

The easiest way to give your child all these vitamins and minerals is via a daily multivitamin. Compare the levels on the packs with the levels that we recommend. In Resources, we list suppliers of good-quality products.

Essential Fat—Oiling the Mental Wheels

Back in the 1980s, the extent of supplementation for children was vitamins and minerals. Today we know that supplementing omega-3 fats is just as important. They not only improve your child's emotional intelligence and behavior, as we'll see in chapter 14, they also keep those mental wheels well oiled and running fast and smoothly.

The levels of omega-3 fats at birth, especially DHA—the brain-building fat—predict intellectual development later in life.[11] And there is overwhelming evidence that supplementing DHA in infants improves the speed of their thinking and other measures of mental performance at ages 3 and 4.[12] So the effects of optimum nutrition during pregnancy and early infancy are long lasting. Although not proven yet, it is highly likely that supplementation with fish oils rich in omega-3s throughout infancy and childhood will maximize a child's intellectual development.

Eating oily coldwater fish is an excellent way of getting more omega-3s into your child's diet, and the chart below shows the amounts of DHA in each type. As we saw in chapter 3, however, be careful to choose fish that is lower in mercury, typically the smaller fish.

Best Fish for Brain Fats

Milligrams of DHA in 3.5 oz (100 g)	
Herring	1,000
Sardines	1,000
Tuna	900
Anchovies	900
Salmon	800
Trout	500

An ideal intake of DHA for your child is on the order of 300 mg to 400 mg a day. So if he is eating 3.5 ounces (100 g) of oily fish (preferably sardines, unsalted anchovies, or herring) three times a week, he'll be doing very well. If your child is new to this type of food, introduce him to it slowly.

Remember that many children will reject a completely new food the first time they encounter it and will often need to try it three or four times to really make up their minds. So don't give up on the first refusal, just ask him to try a little on each occasion. Believe it or not, children in Britain who have been raised eating these foods willingly eat sardines or smoked herring on toast for breakfast! Alternatively, your child can take a supplement of fish oils containing DHA. A good one can provide up to 200 mg.

The best source of all, at least for babies, is breast milk. It's naturally rich in DHA, particularly if the mother is eating fish or flaxseeds. Breast-fed babies not only have higher IQs ten years down the road, and better results in exams, they also have fewer mental health problems.[13]

In chapters 15 and 16 we'll show you some of the extraordinary results already achieved in children with dyslexia, ADHD, and other learning difficulties. You'll also learn how EPA, another kind of omega-3 fat abundant in fish oil, seems to help these children more than DHA. Therefore, we recommend that you supplement both DHA and EPA.

The Ideal Daily Supplement Program, in Milligrams: Omega-3s and Omega-6s

Age	Less than 1	1	2	3–4	5–6	7–8	9–11
Essential Fats							
GLA	50	75	95	110	135	135	135
EPA	100	175	250	300	350	350	350
DHA	100	140	175	200	225	225	225

Fish oils are the best way of supplementing omega-3s, but they're not to everyone's liking. However, nowadays there are many supplements, gels, oils, and capsules cleverly flavored to entice your child into developing the vital habit of supplementing fish oils every day.

Because oily fish can contain mercury, as we've pointed out, the fish oil supplements you give your child should be purified to be mercury free. Choosing a good quality supplement is therefore of the utmost importance.

So the first steps to maximizing your child's IQ are the following:

- Ensure an optimum intake of vitamins and minerals, both from diet and supplements, by giving your child a high-strength children's multivitamin and mineral supplement every day, not one based solely on the RDAs. (Also see chapter 26.)
- Optimize your child's intake of essential fats, especially omega-3 fats, by giving her flaxseeds, oily fish, and/or fish oil supplements every day.

These are the basics. But there's still plenty more that you can do to enhance your child's all-around intelligence, coming up in the next three chapters.

Chapter 12

Developing Concentration and a Sharp Memory

As a parent, you'll have seen at least one child who can't sit still, fidgets all the time, and seems to lack a normal attention span. In fact, attention deficit has become one of the most common problems afflicting today's children. Being able to stay focused on a task, project, or piece of schoolwork is a key part of maximizing a child's abilities. As we saw in the last chapter, achieving optimum nutrition through diet and supplements raises IQ partly because children concentrate better. Vitamins, however, aren't the key factor for concentration. It's sugar—or more precisely, blood sugar balance.

KEY TO CONCENTRATION— BLOOD SUGAR BALANCE

As we saw in chapter 2, keeping an even blood sugar level is critical to intelligence because, more than anything else, it affects your child's ability to concentrate over long periods of time.

Why so? In a nutshell, it all comes down to the brain's fuel, glucose, the sugar derived from the carbohydrates we eat. If over time your child eats too much of the wrong kind of carbohydrates, such as candy and refined starchy foods, his blood and brain sugar levels start yo-yoing. When his blood sugar suddenly dips, his concentration can wander, and any aggressive behavior can get worse.[1]

This reaction is why it is absolutely vital that your child eats a wholesome breakfast and doesn't snack on sugary foods and drinks. A recent school survey found that almost two-thirds (65 percent) of pupils eat candy, chocolate bars, or cookies at least once a day; 64 percent drink soft drinks that contain sugar; and 31 percent eat french fries or potato chips. All of these give your child a rush of sugar to his brain, followed abruptly by a sugar crash and poor concentration.

Aptos Middle School in San Francisco took this message to heart and removed all sugary drinks from its vending machines. They also banned all refined carbohydrate snacks and foods, such as french fries, from the cafeteria. Since the nutrition changes were put into place, administrators and teachers report better student behavior after lunch, fewer afternoon visits to the counseling office, less litter in the schoolyard, and more students sitting down to eat. The school also reported higher scores on standardized tests. Their motto now? "No empty calories!"

Queensbury School in Dunstable, Bedfordshire, was the first British school to follow suit. The school recently removed all sodas, chips, and candy from its vending machines and started to provide free drinking water. Nigel Hill, the headmaster, said, "We took the ethical decision that is facing thousands of schools. Do you put students' health first, or the money you can make from selling them chocolate and sodas?" One year later, deputy head Karen Hayward, who is in charge of the project, told us that removing the soda machine was literally the best decision the school had ever made. There has been a definite improvement, especially in pupils with ADHD-type problems.

The Importance of Eating Breakfast

Other schools have developed campaigns to encourage children who don't eat breakfast to get into the habit of having it. If that sounds peculiar to you because your child always leaves the house energized by a plate of eggs or a bowl of oatmeal, you should know that many children start the school day hungry. But those who do eat breakfast have much better concentration and attention spans, according to a number of studies.[2]

Breakfast should become a golden rule in any household, but it's equally important that the breakfast is a nourishing one. So, if your child eats breakfast at school, check out what's available. Doughnuts and sugary cereals, for instance, don't constitute a good breakfast at all.

The best breakfast is a low-GL one. As we saw in chapter 2, low-GL carbohydrates keep your child's blood sugar even. Cereal is an easy and deservedly popular breakfast choice, but one with a number of pitfalls—few store-bought cereals are low-GL. Let's look at the options in the chart below.

Glycemic Load of Breakfast Cereals

Item	Serving size (in oz)	GL per serving
Oatmeal made from rolled oats	1.1	2
Muesli, gluten-free	1.1	7
All-Bran	1.1	9
Muesli, Natural	1.1	11
Raisin Bran (Kellogg's)	1.1	12
Bran Flakes	1.1	13
Special K (Kellogg's)	1.1	14
Cheerios	1.1	15
Frosted Flakes (Kellogg's)	1.1	15
Weetabix	1.1	16
Grapenuts (Kraft)	1.1	16
Shredded Wheat (Nabisco)	1.1	17
Rice Krispies (Kellogg's)	1.1	22
Cornflakes (Kellogg's)	1.1	24

Source: The GL values of foods listed here are derived from research published by K. Foster-Powell, S. H. Holt, and J. C. Brand-Miller, "International Table of Glycemic Index and Glycemic Load Values," *American Journal of Clinical Nutrition* 76, no. 1 (2002): 5–56.

The goal is for breakfast to be no more than 10 GL, including added fruit—a score somewhat dependent on your child's age and size. So ideally, the cereal part should be no more than 5 GL. As you can see, that rules out almost every branded cereal.

The best breakfast cereal option by far is rolled oats, which can be eaten cooked and hot or raw and cold, sweetened with fresh fruit. Alternatively, you could make your own low-GL muesli with rolled oats, seeds, nuts, and oat bran and sweeten your child's daily portion with fresh fruit.

But you don't have to give your child cereal. As an alternative, serve high-protein, low-GL, and thoroughly delectable options such as eggs served with whole-grain toast or lox with cream cheese on a whole-grain bagel. (See chapter 24 for other practical and delicious breakfasts.)

Grazing the Low-GL Way

Eating low-GL, slow-releasing carbohydrates and grazing, not gorging, is the best way to avoid blood sugar dips. So it's good to encourage whole-some snacking from the start by having a bountiful bowl of fruit available at all times. The best fruits are apples, pears, peaches, and any berries, from strawberries to blueberries. Provided your child is not too young to be nibbling on nuts or seeds, a handful of pumpkinseeds, sunflower seeds, or almonds is also a great snack. Ideally, look for seeds and nuts that are raw and unsalted. Toasted and salted nuts and seeds are not as nutritious, but they're a good alternative to a bag of potato chips, for instance. Try lightly toasting your own seeds at home—they are especially delicious with a sprinkling of tamari (similar to soy sauce). As far as school is concerned, you can always send your child off armed with an apple and a bag of nuts and seeds.

Other good snacks are oatcake crackers, available at some grocery stores, specialty markets, and online (look for the brand name Nairn's). Choose oatcake crackers that are sugar free, because these have the lowest GL score. Although they do contain sugar, oat cookies make a good treat because they are lower GL due to the use of oats instead of wheat flour. It's also an excellent idea to have a nonsugary spread, such as unsweetened peanut or any other nut butter, in your pantry. A teaspoon spread on an oatcake cracker makes for a delicious, sustaining, and wholesome snack.

Farewell to the Fizz

The worst offenders, as far as sugar is concerned, are sodas. A two-liter bottle of cola contains more than 40 teaspoons of sugar! Most of these drinks are best avoided. The best to encourage is water: if a child is brought up drinking water when thirsty, that is what he'll drink. Of all the fruit juices, apple, pear, and orange are best, but make sure you pick 100 percent fresh fruit juices, dilute by at least half with water, and don't make it a staple. Avoid products called "fruit juice drinks": these inevitably contain added sugar.

NATURAL MEMORY BOOSTERS

Concentration is one thing, but once your child has finished a task, what about his recall of it? Memory is vital in school and beyond. Let's look at which nutrients are key in this context.

Phosphatidylcholine

The main brain chemical involved in memory is acetylcholine. As we saw in chapter 4, this is derived from phosphatidylcholine (PC), a phospholipid in foods.

The richest dietary sources of phosphatidylcholine are egg yolks and fish, especially sardines. A child needs about 500 to 1,000 mg of phosphatidylcholine a day to maximize mental function. Most lecithin contains about 20 percent phosphatidylcholine, so your child would need 2.5 to 5 g of lecithin a day.

However, choline isn't the only substance you need to make more acetylcholine. Vitamin B5 (pantothenic acid) is essential for the formation of acetylcholine in the body, as are vitamins B1, B12, and C. So memories are also made of a good multivitamin.

In chapter 4, we saw how recent research reveals that taking choline during pregnancy can result in offspring with "superbrains."[3] But supplementing choline later on helps children and adults alike. Dr. Ladd and colleagues at the West Valley College in Saratoga, California, gave eighty students a single 25 g dose of phosphatidylcholine and found a significant improvement in memory ninety minutes later, most likely due to the improved responses of slow learners.[4] If you combine choline with other "smart" nutrients such as pyroglutamate (discussed below), you can achieve the same memory-boosting effect at lower amounts.

Phosphatidylserine

Phosphatidylserine or PS—which like PC is found in eggs and organ meats—is another phospholipid essential to memory. Along with essential fats and protein, PS is one of the main building materials in the "docking ports" on neurons—the receptor sites where neurotransmitters latch on to deliver their messages. As such, PS is very important to the smooth working of your child's brain.

DMAE

DMAE, or dimethylaminoethanol, (again, sardines are a rich source) is a precursor of choline that crosses much more easily from the blood into brain cells, accelerating the brain's production of acetylcholine. It reduces anxiety, stops the mind racing, improves concentration, promotes learning, and acts as a mild brain stimulant.

Slight chemical variations of DMAE have been marketed as the drug Deaner or Deanol, which may be effective in helping children with learning problems, ADHD, and memory and behavior problems.

The ideal dose for memory enhancement is 100 mg for children under seven, and up to 500 mg for teenagers, taken in the morning or midday, not last thing in the evening. (Too much can overstimulate and is therefore not recommended for people diagnosed with schizophrenia, mania, or epilepsy.) Don't expect immediate results. DMAE can take two to three weeks to work, but it's worth waiting for.

Glutamine and Pyroglutamate—Amazing Brain Fuel

While acetylcholine is the major player as far as memory is concerned, many neurotransmitters are also involved. Some stimulate mental processes, while others prevent information overload. A good balance works best.

For example, the stimulating neurotransmitter GABA, which is made from the amino acid glutamine, helps forge links between memories and calms down an overexcited nervous system. However, a slight variation in this key memory molecule, called glutamate, can literally overexcite neurons to death if there is too much of it free or unbound in the bloodstream. (This action is how MSG, or monosodium glutamate, turns up the volume on tastes but can be a bad thing in large quantities.) Another form of this amino acid, pyroglutamate, greatly enhances learning. Pyroglutamate is found in many foods, including fish, dairy products, fruits, and vegetables.

Here are the three ways pyroglutamate helps improve your memory and mental alertness:

- Increases acetylcholine production
- Boosts the number of receptors for acetylcholine
- Improves communication between the left and right hemispheres of the brain

So it improves the brain's "talking and listening," plus cooperation between the two hemispheres. As a result, learning, memory, concentration, and reflex speed will all benefit.

Glutamine is the most abundant amino acid in the cerebrospinal fluid surrounding the brain. It can be used directly as fuel for the brain and has been shown to enhance mood and mental performance and decrease addictive tendencies.[5] In studies designed to test whether glutamine is safe in large doses, researchers from Brigham and Women's Hospital in Boston gave healthy volunteers between 40 and 60 g a day. Not only was it shown to be safe, but one of the side effects was an enhanced ability to solve problems on continuous performance tests. This study was only five days long, showing that glutamine has an immediate effect, and possibly a greater effect over time.[6]

Glutamine is an important nutrient for the brain, and there is good logic to adding 500 mg to 1,000 mg, depending on age, to your child's daily supplement program, especially if he is having learning problems. Don't give glutamine to an autistic child unless under the supervision of a nutritionist, as some autistic children's bodies cannot process it. Glutamine can be bought in powder form; some supplements contain either glutamine or pyroglutamate. As with all the other brain nutrients we've discussed in this chapter—DMAE, phospatidylcholine, phospatidylserine, and pyroglutamate—it's best taken in the morning as it has a stimulative effect on your child's mental function.

So here are a number of simple steps you can take to improve your child's concentration and memory:

- Always give your child a wholesome, low-GL breakfast.
- Encourage snacking on fruit, nuts, seeds, oatcake crackers, or—occasionally—oat cookies.
- Avoid sugary drinks, choosing water and natural juices diluted by at least half instead.
- Add 1 level teaspoon of lecithin high in phosphatidylcholine to your child's cereal each morning, or 2 teaspoons of regular lecithin.
- Alternatively, consider giving your child a supplement that contains a combination of the brain food nutrients listed above—phosphatidylcholine, phosphatidylserine, DMAE, and pyroglutamate.

Chapter 13

Revving Up
Reading and Writing

At the age of five, some kids are just learning their letters and others are reading Hans Christian Andersen—and there are major differences, too, in their progress with pencil and paper. All this is perfectly natural. When it comes to reading and writing, children develop at their own pace; they all take a different length of time and have a different natural aptitude for these vital skills. There can be a gender difference, too, as boys often develop later in this regard.

That said, if your child struggles with reading or writing and is behind in school, you may be able to help her by improving her nutrition.

Reece is a case in point. As he was behind in school, Reece decided he didn't like reading. He also couldn't sit still for long. His mother had taken him to a psychologist, but that hadn't helped. As part of a TV trial for a British morning television program, we encouraged Reece and his mother to carry out a one-week experiment. Reece was to be given ground seeds on his cereal and more fish (for essential fats), less meat, no sugar or foods with chemical additives, and a special drink called Optio, which is the equivalent of a multivitamin and mineral in fruit juice.

On the next page, you can see an example of Reece's handwriting before the changes to his diet, and one week after. Not only did he write one and a half pages in the same length of time, compared to four lines before the diet, but his handwriting also improved dramatically. His mother, who was skeptical about the trial, said:

I thought that nothing could calm this child down. He was very fidgety, he was hard to get into bed, hyperactive and constantly on the go, and with occasional tantrums. Now he's a completely different child. He's a lot calmer, and he wants to do more in school. In two weeks, his reading has gone up a level. He doesn't get so overexcited, and he's much nicer to be with. We are definitely going to stick with the diet.

At the end of the first month, Reece's reading level had gone up a year! Now he loves reading, and his writing is improving by leaps and bounds.

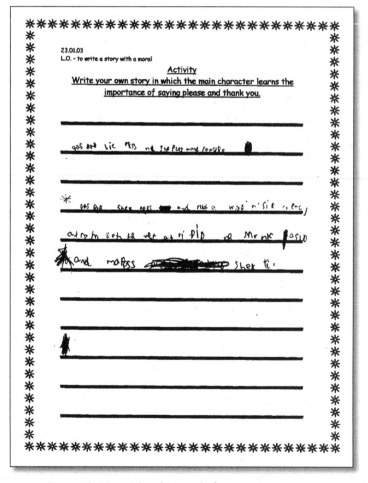

Figure 13. Reece's handwriting before optimum nutrition

Reading and writing problems are often due to perceptual difficulties. One of the first things to rule out is near- or far-sightedness. Often children who struggle to read and write simply have poor eyesight. Improving their eyesight with natural vision improvement methods such as the Bates method, which involves a variety of eye exercises, can bring considerable improvement. Alternatively, get them tested for glasses. However, just as often the problem lies not in the ability of the eyes to focus, but in the ability of the brain to process the information correctly.

An extreme example of this is dyslexia, which we cover in detail in chapter 15. If you are concerned that your child might have dyslexia and know that there's a history of literacy difficulties in your family, complete

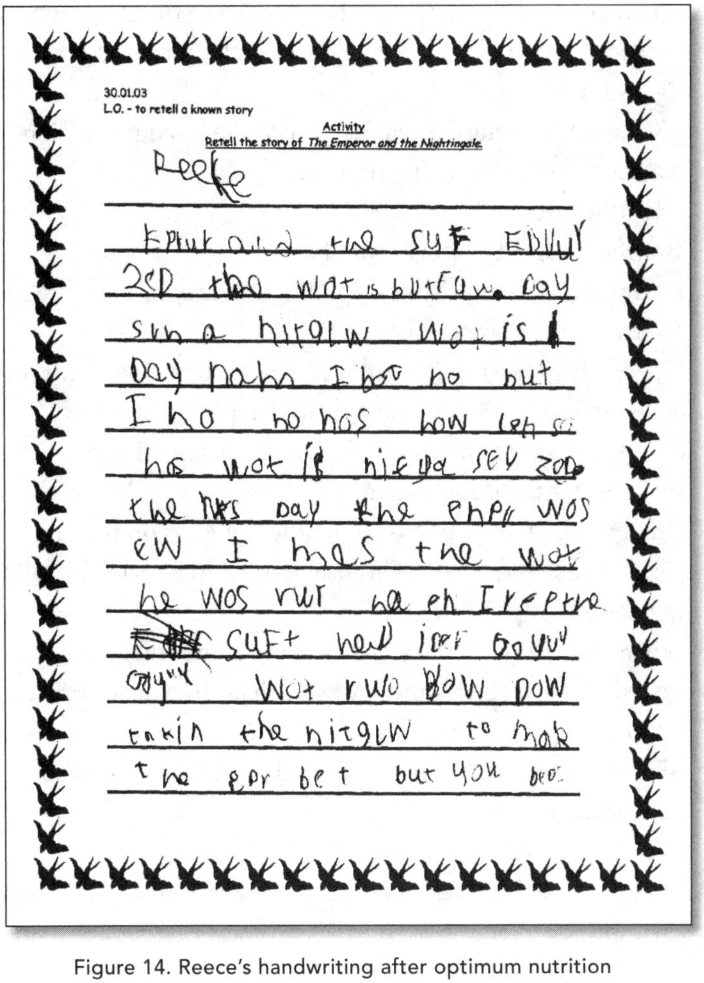

Figure 14. Reece's handwriting after optimum nutrition

the Dyslexia Check below. To answer some of the questions, you may need to see your child in the classroom setting, and/or consult her teacher.

Dyslexia Check

Is your child:

- ❏ A relatively late speaker compared to other children of her age?
- ❏ Good at things that have a strong visual element, but inexplicably poor in other set tasks?
- ❏ Showing evidence of laterality confusion? Ask which hand she writes with, which foot she kicks a ball with, and which eye she uses to look through a cardboard tube. Hand her your watch—which eye does she hold it up to? Does everything happen with the same side or are some things done left-sided and others right-sided?
- ❏ Able to follow a number of instructions in a sequence? For instance, "Go to the living room and get my slippers, then bring them to me."
- ❏ Writing reversed letters or numbers?
- ❏ Having particular difficulty with literacy or one area of literacy, such as spelling or reading?
- ❏ Noticeably inconsistent when reading—recognizing words, then being unable to read the same word later in the day/book/page?
- ❏ Not able to spot words spelled correctly when offered a range of spellings for the same word?
- ❏ Often spelling the same word in different ways on the same page? And if asked the difference between the various spellings, can she identify them?
- ❏ When engaged in literacy tasks, taking a noticeably different time to do them than other tasks, such as drawing or practical activities?
- ❏ Able to give an answer orally or read out a story, but producing little when asked to write it?
- ❏ Described by others as clumsy?
- ❏ Not able to add rhyming or alliterative words to a sequence of rhyming or alliterative words?

❑ Using a much easier reading book than most of her close friends?

❑ In a much lower spelling group than her close friends?

❑ Showing a marked difference compared to the rest of her class during note taking or a copying activity?

❑ Showing a noticeable improvement in work output if given help with planning her work?

❑ Producing more work, and generally seeming much happier in school, if taught strategies to develop sequencing skills?

❑ Beginning to resist writing because she is bad at it?

❑ Looking up at the board during a copying activity much more often than the children around her (suggesting a weak short-term visual memory)?

❑ Responding to a handwriting development program?

❑ Losing confidence over time in an educational setting?

❑ Complaining that the words move around on the page when she is trying to read?

Check the box for each "yes" answer. If you check a lot of "yes" boxes, it's best to see an educational psychologist, who can check out if your child has dyslexia.

THE EYES HAVE IT—OMEGA-3S AND VITAMIN A

Because visual acuity and the ability of the brain to process information from the eye are central to reading and writing, ensuring the eyes and brain are optimally nourished is important if your child is struggling with these skills. And when it comes to that, oily fish and carrots are the dynamic duo.

While we've now seen how the brain is rich in the omega-3 fats some oily fish are positively swimming in, there is also a concentration of these essential fats in the eyes, along with vitamin A. In fact, so vital is vitamin A to vision that its name, retinol, is a direct reference to its role in keeping the retina working properly. (Retinol is the animal form of vitamin A, found in meat, fish, and eggs; beta-carotene, the vegetable form, is converted into retinol in the body.)

Some fish oil supplements—notably cod liver oil—contain both vitamin A as retinol and omega-3 fats, so if you suspect your child's problems with reading or writing are caused by vision problems, you could try giving her this kind of supplement for a month. Some children will take it right off the spoon, or if they're old enough a capsule might be more palatable. Otherwise, try mixing it into her food, although the taste can difficult to mask.

The ideal amount of omega-3, and most specifically DHA and EPA, is given on page 208. With vitamin A, it is vital to know safe limits, as it is one of the few vitamins that can be stored in the body and very large amounts may cause problems.

During pregnancy, for instance, a woman taking more than 5,000 mcg (16,500 IU) of vitamin A a day may increase the risk of birth defects in her child. For your child, the ideal amount is much less than this—between 500 mcg (1,650 IU) and 2,000 mcg (6,600 IU), depending on your child's age (see page 207). The table below shows how much your child would need to eat to achieve 500 mcg (1,650 IU).

Vitamin A in Foods

Type of food	Amount giving 500 mcg (1,650 IU) of vitamin A (as retinol)
Liver	0.1 oz (3 g)
Cream cheese	4 oz (110 g)
Kidney	4.5 oz (130 g)
Cheddar cheese	5.5 oz (160 g)
Whole milk	5.5 oz (160 g)
Parmesan cheese	8.5 oz (240 g)
Mackerel	31 oz (900 g)
Chicken	56 oz (1.6 kg)
Egg	6 large eggs
Butter	11 tablespoons

Of course, no one is going to eat that much egg, butter, mackerel, or chicken at one sitting, but it's important to know how much vitamin A your child's food contains so you can balance that out with all other sources of vitamin A. Most multivitamins will contain some retinol, usually about

500 mcg (1,650 IU). Cod liver oil capsules vary considerably, however, so do check the label—most will provide between 500 mcg (1,650 IU) and 1,000 mcg (3,300 IU) per capsule.

You'll need to ensure that the combination of food, supplements, and fish oil capsules, added up, doesn't exceed double the optimum daily supplemental amount of vitamin A according to your child's age, shown on page 207. However, do make sure your child is getting both omega-3s and vitamin A.

PESTICIDES—BAD NEWS FOR THE EYES

When the eye is processing visual information, it turns vitamin A into rhodopsin, a light-sensitive pigment. Light reaching rhodopsin reacts with it, after which the pigment undergoes a cycle of changes that, effectively, recycles it so it turns back into rhodopsin. This cycle is particularly important for black and white vision, which is for the most part what we use at night—hence your grandmother always telling you carrots help you see in the dark.

Organophosphate pesticides and herbicides, now being phased out in most developed countries but still used widely in developing countries, block this conversion. While this is unlikely to be a significant factor in your child's visual ability, it does highlight why it is so important to keep our children free from such chemicals—so keep choosing organic food whenever you can (see chapter 8).

There are several simple steps you can take to support your child's reading and writing:

- Ensure an optimum intake of vitamin A from food, supplements, and fish oil capsules.
- Optimize your child's intake of essential fats, especially omega-3s, by giving her flaxseeds, oily fish, and/or fish oil supplements every day.
- Keep your child chemical free by choosing organic food whenever possible.

Chapter 14

Enhancing Mood
and Behavior

Childhood is supposed to be a joyful time, but there is a danger here of succumbing to a stereotype. It simply doesn't always pan out that way. From the child's point of view, day-to-day life often falls far short of the ideal. Many are no strangers to sadness, boredom, ennui, irritability, and anger.

According to research at two British universities, the University of London and Warwick University, the incidence of depression among young people has doubled over the past twelve years. Exact figures for the United States are difficult to come by, but indications are that incidence has been steadily increasing for the past couple of decades. The use of SSRI antidepressant medication was also showing a growing trend until 2004. After the release of data that showed an increased tendency to suicidal thoughts and behavior in children and adolescents taking this class of antidepressants, the FDA required manufacturers to strengthen warnings of these potential side effects.[1] Subsequently, the use of this class of medication in children has seen a significant decline both in the United States and abroad.

Much better solutions than this are at hand. So if your child is frequently sad or cries a lot, doesn't enjoy or participate in activities, is always bored, has low self-esteem, or is irritable, angry, hostile to others, or self-destructive, you can help him. There are two avenues to explore—psychological and biochemical. But as we'll see, they're intimately intertwined.

GETTING TO THE ROOT OF UNHAPPINESS

Conventionally, anger is not an emotion adults are allowed to express, much less children. Some kids—angry at something happening in school, with their friends, or at home—bottle it up as depression. Although you, as a parent, can help tremendously, every child also benefits from having an open, sympathetic adult other than his parents to talk to, guide him, and help him find solutions to his problems.

One of the greatest unrecognized truths is the role of nutrition in the psychological health of our children. Ensuring your child is optimally nourished will not only improve his mood, but also give him the energy and motivation to deal with life's inevitable ups and downs. Few child psychotherapists and pediatricians recognize how much better their results would be if they helped children tune up their brain biochemistry.

There are a number of common imbalances connected to nutrition that can worsen a child's mood and motivation, some of which will already be familiar:

- Blood sugar imbalances (often associated with excessive sugar and caffeine intake)
- Deficiencies of nutrients (vitamin B3, B6, B12, and C, folate, zinc, magnesium, and essential fats)
- Deficiencies of tryptophan and tyrosine (precursors of neurotransmitters)
- Allergies and sensitivities

Poor control of blood glucose levels is a causative factor in low mood, yet it is a relatively simple aspect of your child's daily routine to fix. As we saw in chapter 2, you can help him here by always providing breakfast, as well as regular meals and snacks composed of natural, unprocessed foods. But what about those key nutrients?

BEATING THE BLUES WITH NUTRITION

Among nutrients, the most promising for improving mood are vitamins B3 and B12 and folic acid, then vitamin B6, zinc, magnesium, and the essential fats (especially omega-3s, which we discussed in detail in chapter 3). The first three are involved in the biochemical process known as methylation, which is critical for balancing the neurotransmitters that keep your child motivated and happy. Improved methylation is also associated with better grades.

The B Connection

Folic acid is found in green leafy vegetables, nuts, seeds, and beans. Far too many children have far too few of these foods, yet their effect can be astounding—as an intriguing study by Bernard Gesch has shown.

Gesch wondered what the effect of giving B vitamins and essential fats to Britain's worst juvenile delinquents would be. After persuading the UK Home Office to allow the first UK double-blind trial on juvenile delinquents in a maximum security prison, he gave them either a multinutrient containing vitamins, minerals, and essential fats, or a placebo. The results, published in the *British Journal of Psychiatry*, showed a staggering 35 percent decrease in acts of aggression in the prisoners eating the multivitamin after only two weeks.[2]

Since prison diets are, if anything, already better than those most of these young people ate at home, this shows just how important optimum nutrition is for reducing violent and deviant behavior. When the trial was over and the supplements were stopped, there was a 40 percent increase in offenses in the prison.

Magnesium—Relaxing Mind and Muscle

Gesch also gave magnesium and zinc to the juvenile delinquents in his study. These two minerals are among the most important for mental health. We've seen how zinc, for instance, helps with problems such as confusion, depression, and slow mental processing. Magnesium has a relaxant effect on both mind and muscles, and deficiencies are very common, manifesting as muscle aches, cramps and spasms, as well an anxiety, irritability and insomnia. Children often have low levels, which can be helped via supplementation.

A child needs between 250 and 500 mg of magnesium a day. Seeds and nuts are rich in magnesium, as are vegetables and fruit, especially dark green leafy vegetables such as chard or spinach. We recommend that children eat these magnesium-rich foods every day and supplement an additional 50 to 100 mg of magnesium. See part 4 for ideas on how to get your child to eat vegetables.

Fats to Fight Depression

We've already encountered omega-3 fish oils in a number of contexts. And as it happens, they are very much part of the equation for happiness. The better a child's blood levels of omega-3 fats, the better his levels of serotonin—the "happy" neurotransmitter—are likely to be. The reason for this is that omega-3 fats help to build the brain's receptor sites for serotonin, as well as improve reception. According to Dr. Joseph Hibbeln, who discovered that fish eaters are less prone to depression, "It's like building more serotonin factories, instead of just increasing the efficiency of the serotonin you have."[3] Many trials have now been published proving that omega-3 fats are highly effective as a treatment for depression.[4] EPA is the top omega-3 for this job.

A case in point is a small-scale study by Dr. Basant Puri from London's Hammersmith Hospital. Puri decided to try ethyl-EPA on one of his patients, a twenty-one-year-old student who had been on a variety of antidepressants to no avail. He had a very low sense of self-esteem, sleeping problems, and little appetite, found it hard to socialize, and often thought of killing himself. After a month of supplemented omega-3 fats, he was no longer having suicidal thoughts and after nine months no longer had any depression.[5]

BALANCING ACT— NEUROTRANSMITTERS AND MOOD

There are often two sides to feeling low—feeling miserable, and feeling apathetic and unmotivated. The most prevalent theory for the cause of these mood states is a brain imbalance in two families of neurotransmitters, the molecules of emotion: serotonin, which influences your mood; and adrenaline and noradrenaline, made from dopamine, which influence your motivation.

But this imbalance isn't just about nutrition. Let's look at some of the other factors in your child's life that could be fueling any unhappiness and apathy he's experiencing.

Stresses and Strains—How Imbalance Sets In

The mad, goal-driven dash of twenty-first-century living can be very stressful for children. Too many children are pressured to perform in a century where the motto is "Be the best." Perhaps living out their parent's dissatisfactions, they go from school to piano lessons to extra coaching, with no time left to simply do nothing, dream, or play.

All this has an inevitable effect on the brain, which produces more and more adrenaline and serotonin in response to the too frequent ups and downs, and numerous stresses and strains. It's akin to the body's production of more and more insulin to even out frequently fluctuating blood sugar levels; this increases a child's need for the building blocks, the amino acids, from which we make these mood-enhancing neurotransmitters. Combine these psychological pressures with the all-too-common poor diet, and too many children go over the edge into low moods and erratic behavior.

Over the last few years, what has been learned about both serotonin, the "happy" neurotransmitter, and adrenaline and noradrenaline, "the motivators," is that there are four main reasons for deficiency in children, in addition to a lack of amino acids:

- Not enough light
- Not enough exercise
- Too much stress
- Not enough cofactor B vitamins, zinc, and magnesium

So if your child is melancholy or depressed, misbehaving, or exhausted; tends to comfort himself with food; and is experiencing disturbed sleep patterns, the chances are that a combination of factors are working together to leave him short on serotonin, noradrenaline, or adrenaline.

How does it happen? Light is very important as a brain stimulator, yet with our increasingly indoor lives most of us don't get enough of it. The difference in light exposure outside and inside is striking. Many of us spend twenty-three out of twenty-four hours a day indoors, exposed to 200 to 500 units (called lux) of light. Compare that to the 20,000 lux of a sunny day and the 7,000 lux of an overcast day. Most of us are simply not exposing ourselves to enough direct sunlight to maximize serotonin production. And, of course, it's worse in winter when the days are shorter, especially in the northern states.

Stress—from exams or bullying, for example—also rapidly reduces serotonin levels and raises adrenaline, leading to burnout. A couch-potato habit can make this worse because physical exercise improves the stress response and reduces the stress-induced depletion of serotonin and adrenaline. Exercise itself is an incredibly powerful mood booster.

The message is that you need to ensure your child has the time and opportunity to exercise and play outdoors for a reasonable length of time daily.

SUPPLEMENTING FOR NEUROTRANSMITTER BALANCE

You might find that your child needs extra help in recovering from difficulties with mood. In these cases, look to supplementation. There are a number of possibilities.

Go for the Right Amino Acids

Serotonin is made from a constituent of protein, the amino acid tryptophan. Dr. Philip Cowen from Oxford University's psychiatry department has proven that if you deprive adults of tryptophan, most experience a worsening of mood and start to show signs of depression within seven hours.[6] Tryptophan is especially abundant in fish, turkey, chicken, cheese, beans, tofu, oats, and eggs. A child's diet, depending on age, needs to contain between 500 mg and 1,000 mg of tryptophan a day, which they can easily achieve by eating one or two of the following meals, each giving 500 mg:

- Oatmeal, soymilk, and two scrambled eggs
- Baked potato with cottage cheese and tuna salad
- Chicken breast, potatoes au gratin, and green beans
- Whole wheat spaghetti with bean, tofu, or meat sauce
- Salmon fillet, quinoa and lentil pilaf, and green salad with yogurt dressing

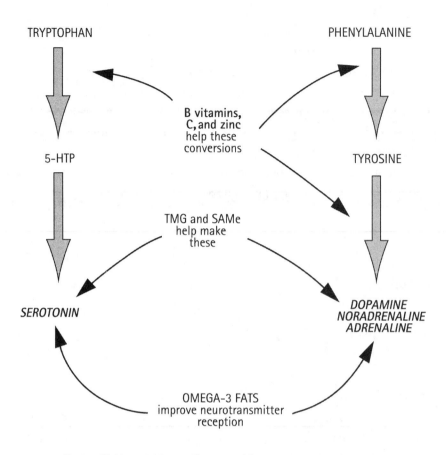

Figure 15. How nutrients affect mood-boosting neurotransmitters

Adrenaline and noradrenaline are made from the amino acids phenylalanine and tyrosine. These are found in protein foods—the same kind that are rich in tryptophan. So ensuring adequate protein intake, as we saw in chapter 5, helps keep your child's mood and motivation positive.

In adult studies, supplementing 5-hydroxytryptophan (5-HTP), the amino acid from which the body makes serotonin, along with tyrosine, the amino acid from which the body makes adrenaline and noradrenaline, has proven highly effective in correcting mood problems.

There have been twenty-seven studies to date giving adults 100 to 900 mg of 5-HTP a day, showing it to be highly effective in restoring a balanced mood, without any significant side effects. The worst that seems to happen is that, with very large doses, some people become nauseated. For children, depending on age, supplement between 20 and 50 mg of 5-HTP. Not only is 5-HTP a highly effective mood booster, much more so than antidepressants, it also has no significant side effects.[7]

Try TMG—The Master Tuner

In Figure 15, you might have noticed two strange-sounding nutrients: TMG (trimethylglycine) and SAMe (S-adenosylmethionine). Both are amino acids that help to keep the brain and nervous system well tuned by donating so-called methyl groups. These are important in the transformation of neurotransmitters. For example, noradrenaline turns into adrenaline by having a methyl group added. This process of adding on methyl groups, and sometimes taking them away, is crucial to the task of keeping the brain in balance.

SAMe is one of the most comprehensively studied natural antidepressants. Over 100 placebo-controlled, double-blind studies show that SAMe is equal to or superior to antidepressants and works faster—most often within a few days (most pharmaceutical antidepressants may take three to six weeks to take effect)—and with few side effects.[8]

While SAMe is classified as a medicine, TMG, the amino acid from which it is made, is a component of food and is especially high in roots and sprouts. So eating carrots, parsnips, beets, turnips, potatoes, and bean sprouts will provide your child with TMG. Although it's not classified as an essential nutrient, we recommend that children eat at least 100 mg a day, which translates to a serving of a root vegetable or sprouts.

To help your child with behavioral problems and low mood, give him supplements with amino acids (5-HTP, phenylalanine or tyrosine, and TMG) together with the B vitamins that help turn them into neurotransmitters (B3, B6, B12, and folic acid). Some children's formulas contain these nutrients, which literally help the brain connect properly.

At the Brain Bio Centre in London, we test children for their blood levels of essential fats, blood platelet levels of serotonin, adrenaline, and noradrenaline, as well as homocysteine, which tells whether a child needs more B vitamins and TMG. From that, we can devise the perfect nutrition program of food and supplements to help him achieve his full potential. To have your child's homocysteine level tested, speak to your doctor. The tests for essential fats and neurotransmitters are more specialized and may be available only from a nutritionist.

> Fourteen-year-old Liam had been expelled from mainstream school for disruptive behavior. His homocysteine score was 24—the average for a ninety-year-old! One month of B vitamins, magnesium, TMG, and omega-3 supplements, along with a low-sugar diet, brought his level down to 9. In his own words:
>
> > *About ten days after starting the diet and the vitamins, I noticed I was less tired in the morning. Now I'm not tired at all when I wake up. I have loads more energy, I'm less bored, I'm concentrating better, and I feel a lot happier. I'm getting on better in school and concentrating better in class. I'm also doing more activities and sports. I feel better, having reduced my homocysteine level. I feel more positive about my future. Since starting the diet, I'm a lot calmer than I used to be and I haven't been in trouble at all. I'm going to stay on the diet for life and keep taking the vitamins. It's brilliant!*

To keep your child's mood, motivation, and behavior good, do the following:

- Give him a diet containing protein-rich foods (fish, meat, eggs, legumes) and TMG-rich foods (root vegetables, sprouts).
- Optimize your child's intake of essential fats, especially omega-3 fats, by giving him flaxseeds, oily fish, and/or fish oil supplements every day.
- Ensure optimum nutrition with a good multivitamin providing all the B vitamins, plus magnesium and zinc.
- If your child is low in energy, mood, or motivation, or is under stress, underperforming, or acting up, give him an additional supplement containing TMG, 5-HTP, and tyrosine or phenylalanine.

PART 3

Solving Problems

A re children today having a kid-life crisis? Mental health problems are very much on the increase in children, from autism and learning difficulties to hyperactivity and aggression. A major reason for these increases is often suboptimum nutrition. In this part of the book, we give you nutritional solutions to these and other problems to help you maximize your child's potential for mental and emotional health and happiness.

Chapter 15

Dyslexia and Dyspraxia— What Works

Nowadays, any child with learning and behavioral problems tends to get put into one of a number of boxes. Is she dyslexic, having problems with words and writing? Is she dyspraxic, having problems with coordination? Does she have attention deficit/hyperactivity disorder (ADHD), the official term for what used to be known as hyperactivity but still denotes poor attention span and concentration and hyperactive behavior?

In most children who have problems with learning or behavior, there are substantial overlaps between these categories. While a minority of children are purely dyslexic, more will show features of two or all three of these conditions in differing degrees of severity. Around half the dyslexic population is likely to be dyspraxic, and vice versa, and the mutual overlap between ADHD and dyslexia/dyspraxia is also around 50 percent.[1] But unfortunately, it's rare to find a diagnosis or treatment that takes these complexities into account. ADHD, for instance, lies firmly in the realm of psychiatry and is usually treated with stimulant medication (see chapter 16).

IS YOUR CHILD AFFECTED?

Children with dyslexia experience specific problems in learning to read and write, sometimes because of subtle variations in visual perception. Difficulties in arithmetic and reading musical notation are also common,

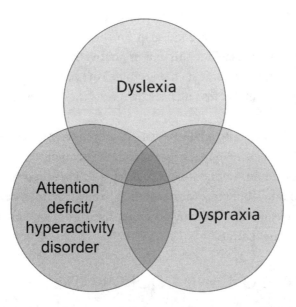

Figure 16. Dyslexia, dyspraxia, and attention deficit/hyperactivity disorder overlap

as are poor working memory, problems with deciphering the sounds of words, and a faulty sense of direction.

Around 5 percent of the population is severely dyslexic, although many more are affected by milder forms of the condition. If you suspect your child might be dyslexic, begin by completing the Dyslexia Check in chapter 13, page 112. Your school should have special needs teachers who can assess your child thoroughly. If your child's school doesn't do this, contact the International Dyslexia Association (see Resources, page 215); they can put you in touch with an educational psychologist who can carry out this assessment.

Getting your child assessed is useful on a number of counts: it helps her become aware that she has a difficulty, allows her to work with a special needs teacher to minimize the problem, and gives her special privileges such as more time for exams and the use of computers in school.

Recent research suggests that pure dyslexia—that is, substantially delayed reading and writing in otherwise bright children—may have to do with a subtle brain difference in how these children perceive the "small sounds," or phonetic building blocks, of words. This perception makes it harder for them to both read and understand word meanings, as they simply don't have a good grip on the basics. Special teaching techniques to compensate for this can dramatically improve your child's reading and writing skills. If such assistance isn't available through your child's school, the International Dyslexia Association can help you locate a teacher.

Less well-known but equally prevalent, dyspraxia involves poor coordination and difficulties in carrying out complex sequenced actions. Children with this condition find it hard to catch a ball, tie their shoelaces, or button their clothes, but more seriously, their handwriting can be extremely difficult to read, and they can experience real difficulties with organization, attention, and concentration.

EAT FOR VISION AND COORDINATION

On top of assessments and tailored teaching, children with dyslexia and dyspraxia can benefit deeply from the right nutrition. Again, it comes down to nutrients that will help the brain and eyes.

Essential Fats—Seeing Is Believing

We discussed the importance of essential fats for proper brain function in chapter 3. Children with dyslexia, dyspraxia, and learning difficulties are very often deficient in these essential fats and/or the nutrients needed to properly utilize them, and the benefits of increasing the intake of these fats have been clearly documented in many studies.[2] A high concentration of essential fats is needed in the eyes before they can manage the very rapid movements associated with vision.

A study of ninety-seven dyslexic children by Dr. Alex Richardson and colleagues at Hammersmith Hospital in London revealed that essential fat deficiency clearly contributes to the severity of dyslexic problems. Those children with the worst essential fat deficiencies showed significantly poorer reading and lower general ability than the nondeficient children.[3]

How do you know if your child is deficient in essential fats? You could start with the Fat Check in chapter 3, page 34. A key indicator is dry skin or eczema, and in a study of sixty children at the Royal London Hospital, Dr. Christine Absolon and colleagues found twice the rate of "psychological disturbance" in children with eczema, compared to those without.[4]

If your child has some of the outward symptoms of essential fat deficiency—rough, dry patches on the skin, cracked lips, dull or dry hair, soft or brittle nails, and excessive thirst—it is fair to say that this could be an underlying factor in learning difficulties she might be experiencing, such as concentration or visual problems, mood swings, disturbed sleep patterns, and in some cases behavioral problems. Dyslexia, dyspraxia, learning difficulties, and ADHD all involve poor nerve cell communications in the brain, and essential fats are crucial in keeping neurons talking to each other.[5]

To test the value of supplementing essential fats in dyspraxia, Dr. Jacqueline Stordy of the University of Surrey, England, gave essential fat supplements containing DHA, EPA, AA, and DGLA to fifteen children whose performance on standardized measures of motor and coordination skills placed them in the bottom 1 percent of the population. After twelve weeks of supplementation, they all showed significant improvements in manual dexterity, ball skills, balance, and parental ratings of their dyspraxic symptoms.[6]

Stordy also assessed the benefit of essential fat supplementation in dyslexia and found that after just four weeks of supplementation with EPA and DHA, night vision and dark adaptation (which are usually very poor in dyslexics) had completely normalized.[7]

Of course, it's just as vital for kids with dyslexia and dyspraxia to avoid fried and hydrogenated fats as to top up their essential fats.

The Copper-Zinc Link

While much of the current research into nutritional solutions for dyslexia and dyspraxia is focusing on essential fats, some scientists are looking at copper, a potentially toxic element reported to be high in dyslexic children.[8] Since zinc and vitamin C are both antagonists of copper, this is a possible explanation for their reported benefits.

Along with the recommendations in chapter 13, we suggest you take the following steps if your child is dyslexic or dyspraxic:

- Ensure she's getting an optimal intake of nutrients from her diet as well as a good-quality multivitamin and mineral supplement with enough zinc.
- Minimize your child's intake of sugar and refined or processed foods, which provide ample calories but few nutrients, and encourage her to eat more nutrient-rich foods.
- Ensure an optimal intake of essential fats from seeds, their cold-pressed oils, and oily fish, plus sufficient antioxidants, especially vitamin E, to protect her from free-radical damage.
- Minimize your child's intake of fried food, processed food, and saturated fat from meat and dairy.

Chapter 16

Drug-Free Solutions for ADHD

It seems incredible, but an estimated 1 in 10 children in the United States is affected by attention deficit/hyperactivity disorder, or ADHD. Children with this condition just can't sit still, have a short attention span and volatile moods, get into fights, and disrupt their classes. They have a hard time in school and at home, performing badly, getting into trouble, and often being shunted from school to school. Untreated, a hyperactive six-year-old might grow up to become a delinquent teenager, getting derailed by drugs and alcohol.

At a cursory glance, ADHD might look like something to be blamed on poor parenting or schooling. But dig more deeply, and a plethora of other potential causative factors emerges: heredity, smoking, alcohol or drug use during their mothers' pregnancy, oxygen deprivation at birth, prenatal trauma, and environmental pollution.

The good news is that, more often than not, children with ADHD have one or more nutritional imbalances. Identifying and correcting these can dramatically improve the children's energy, focus, concentration, and behavior.

> Eight-year-old Richard is a case in point. Diagnosed with ADHD, he was out of control, and his parents were at their wits' end. Richard had also been constipated his entire life. Through biochemical testing at the Brain Bio Centre, we found that he was allergic to dairy products and eggs and was very deficient in

magnesium. Dietary analysis revealed that he took in excessive amounts of sugar every day. We recommended cutting down his sugar intake significantly, cutting out dairy and egg products, and supplementing magnesium and omega-3 essential fats. Within three months, his parents reported that Richard had calmed down considerably and had become much more manageable. His constipation had also disappeared.

It can be difficult to draw the line between the behavior of a child that is within the normal limits of high energy, and abnormally active behavior. Use the list below to assess your child, scoring 2 if a symptom is severe, 1 if moderate, and 0 if not present.

Hyperactivity Check

Is your child:

_____ Overactive?
_____ Prone to leave projects unfinished?
_____ Fidgety?
_____ Wearing out toys, furniture, etc.?
_____ Unable to sit still at meals?
_____ Uninterested in staying with games?
_____ Too talkative?
_____ Failing to follow directions?
_____ Clumsy?
_____ Fighting with other children?
_____ Unpredictable?
_____ Teasing?
_____ Unable to respond to discipline?
_____ Getting into things?
_____ Displaying speech problems?
_____ Having temper tantrums?
_____ Unable to listen to a story to the end?
_____ Defiant?
_____ Hard to get to bed?
_____ Irritable?

_____ Reckless?

_____ Unpopular with peers?

_____ Impatient?

_____ Lying?

_____ Accident-prone?

_____ Wetting the bed?

_____ Destructive?

A score below 12 is normal. If it's higher, read on to discover workable nutritional strategies.

EAT TO CALM DOWN

If your child has ADHD and is eating poorly, the way is clear: you'll need to take a very close look at the amount of refined carbohydrates, harmful trans fats, and other problem foods he's consuming, look at what's missing, and provide a menu designed to calm him down.

Show Sugar the Door

In chapter 2, we saw how vital balanced blood sugar levels are to mental health and advocated a low- or no-sugar diet. A diet high in refined carbohydrates is not good for anyone, but in some children eating sweets seems to promote hyperactivity and aggression.

Essentially, if you feed your child rocket fuel (that is, sugar and caffeine), don't be surprised if his behavior is out of control. Even so-called normal children can become uncontrollable after a sugarfest. Dietary studies do consistently reveal that hyperactive children eat more sugar than other children, and reducing sugar has been found to halve disciplinary actions in juvenile offenders.[1]

Other research has confirmed that the problem is not sugar itself, but the forms it comes in, the absence of a well-balanced diet overall, and abnormal glucose metabolism. A study of 265 hyperactive children found that more than three-quarters of them displayed abnormal glucose tolerance; that is, their bodies were less able to handle sugar intake and maintain balanced blood sugar levels.[2]

In any case, when children regularly snack on refined carbohydrates, candy, chocolate, sodas, juices, and little or no fiber to slow glucose absorption, the levels of glucose in their blood will seesaw continually and trigger wild fluctuations in their levels of activity, concentration, focus, and behavior. These, of course, are also the symptoms of ADHD. The initial calm that sometimes sets in after children eat refined carbohydrates may well be a short-lived normalization of blood sugar levels from a hypoglycemic (low blood sugar) state, during which the brain—including those parts of it that control behavior—was starved of fuel.

Since children with hyperactivity and ADHD seem particularly sensitive to sugar, it's recommended that you remove all forms of refined sugar and any foods that contain it from your child's diet, including processed juices and juice drinks—these deliver a big shot of sugar very quickly. Replace these with water or diluted fresh juice, whole foods and complex carbohydrates such as brown rice and other whole grains, oats, lentils, beans, quinoa, and vegetables, which should be eaten throughout the day. Three substantial meals and several snacks will keep blood sugar trickling in slowly and evenly.

To further slow the progress of glucose into his bloodstream, you should ensure that your child's intake of carbohydrates is balanced with protein, so that he eats half as much protein as carbohydrates at every meal and snack. For instance, give him a handful of seeds and nuts with a piece of fruit, or have chicken or fish with rice for dinner.

Pump Up the Essential Fats

As we saw in chapter 12, essential fats are crucial for concentration. Omega-3s in particular have a clearly calming effect on many children with hyperactivity and ADHD. And many children with ADHD, like those with dyslexia, have visible symptoms of essential fat deficiency, such as excessive thirst, dry skin, eczema, and asthma.

It is also interesting that boys, whose requirement for essential fats is much higher than girls', are also much more likely to have ADHD: four out of five sufferers are male. Researchers have theorized that children with ADHD may be deficient in essential fats not just because their dietary intake from foods such as seeds and nuts is inadequate (though this is not uncommon), but also because their need is higher, their absorption is poor, or they are unable to effectively convert these fats into EPA and DHA, and from DHA into prostaglandins, which are also important for brain function.[3] Children with ADHD may show no physical signs of deficiency, such as dry hair and skin and frequent thirst and urination, yet still experience behavioral benefits from supplementing the essential fats.[4]

So it's of interest that the conversion of essential fats can be inhibited by most of the foods that cause symptoms in children with ADHD, such as wheat, dairy, and foods containing salicylates. (More on salicylates later in this chapter.) This conversion is also hindered by deficiencies of the various vitamins and minerals that help the enzymes driving these conversions— vitamin B3 (niacin), B6, C, biotin, zinc, and magnesium. Zinc deficiency is common in children with ADHD.

Research carried out at Purdue University, Indiana, confirmed that children with ADHD have an inadequate intake of the nutrients required for the conversion of essential fats into prostaglandins and have lower levels of EPA, DHA, and AA than children without ADHD.[5] Supplementation with all these omega-3 essential fats, preconverted, along with the omega-6 essential fat GLA, reduced ADHD symptoms such as anxiety, attention difficulties, and general behavior problems.[6]

An Australian study examined the effect of both omega-3 and omega-6 supplements on the behavior of 132 children with ADHD aged seven to twelve. Significant improvement in hyperactivity, attention, and impulsiveness were seen in the children taking the supplements when compared with the control group of children who were given a placebo.[7]

Research at Oxford University has proven the value of these essential fats in a double-blind trial involving forty-one children aged eight to twelve years who had ADHD symptoms and specific learning difficulties. Those children receiving extra essential fats in supplements were both behaving and learning better within twelve weeks.[8] The case study below, courtesy of the Hyperactive Children's Support Group in the UK, is revealing in this context.

> Six-year-old Stephen had a history of hyperactivity, with severely disturbed sleep and disruptive behavior at home and in school. Threatened with expulsion from school because of his impossible behavior, his parents were given two weeks to improve

matters. They contacted the Hyperactive Children's Support Group, and evening primrose oil was suggested. Since Stephen was too young for capsules and wouldn't swallow the oil from a spoon, a dose of 1.5 g was rubbed into his skin morning and evening. The school was unaware of this, but after five days the teacher telephoned the mother to say that never, in thirty years of teaching, had she seen such a dramatic change in a child's behavior.

After three weeks, the evening primrose oil was stopped, and one week later the school again complained. The oil was then reintroduced, and again its effect clearly showed in Stephen's improved behavior. It's worth noting that rubbing oil on the skin is not nearly as effective as taking it by mouth, because only a small percentage of it makes it into the body—so Stephen's story is all the more remarkable.

Many children do not eat rich sources of omega-3 essential fats and could benefit from eating more oily fish (wild or organic salmon, sardines, herring, anchovies, mackerel, fresh tuna) and seeds such as flax, hemp, sunflower, and pumpkin or their cold-pressed oils. It is also important to replace foods known to hinder the conversion of essential fats to prostaglandins—such as deep-fried foods—while supplementing the nutrients needed for the conversion, such as B vitamins and zinc, as discussed above.

Sort Out the Allergies

Of all the avenues so far explored, the link between hyperactivity and food sensitivity is the most established and worthy of pursuit in any child showing signs of ADHD.

A study by Dr. Joseph Bellanti of Georgetown University in Washington, DC, found that hyperactive children are seven times more likely to have food allergies than other children. According to his research, 56 percent of hyperactive children aged seven to ten tested positive for food allergies, compared to less than 8 percent of nonhyperactive children. A separate investigation by the Hyperactive Children's Support Group found that 89 percent of children with ADHD reacted to food colorings, 72 percent to flavorings, 60 percent to MSG, 45 percent to all synthetic additives, 50 percent to cow's milk, 60 percent to chocolate, and 40 percent to oranges.[9] (For more on food additives, see chapter 8.)

Other substances often found to induce behavioral changes are wheat, corn, yeast, soy, peanuts, and eggs.[10] Symptoms strongly linked to allergy include nasal problems and excessive mucus, ear infections, facial swelling and discoloration around the eyes, tonsillitis, digestive problems, bad breath, eczema, asthma, headaches, and bed-wetting. (See chapter 9 for more details on identifying and eliminating food allergies in your child.)

Up to 90 percent of hyperactive children benefit from eliminating foods that contain artificial colors, flavors, and preservatives; processed and manufactured foods; and culprit foods identified by either an exclusion diet or a blood test.[11] Some parents have also reported success with the Feingold diet, removing not only all artificial additives but also foods that naturally contain compounds called salicylates.

Researchers at the University of Sydney in Australia found that three-quarters of eighty-six children with ADHD reacted adversely to foods containing salicylates.[12] These include prunes, raisins, raspberries, almonds, apricots, canned cherries, black currants, oranges, strawberries, grapes, ketchup, plums, cucumbers, and most types of apples. As the list of foods containing salicylates is very long and contains many otherwise nutritious foods, cutting them all out should be considered only as a secondary course of action and must be carefully planned and monitored by a nutritional therapist.

Understanding how a low-salicylate diet helps hyperactive children does offer a useful alternative to such a drastic course of action. Salicylates inhibit the conversion and utilization of essential fats, which we know are often low in hyperactive children. So instead of avoiding salicylates, it may help to simply increase the supply of essential fats, and as we've seen, that has indeed been shown to work.

Fix the Deficiencies

As we've now seen abundantly, studies have shown that academic performance improves and behavioral problems diminish significantly when children are given nutritional supplements. Although it is unlikely, on the basis of the studies to date, that ADHD is purely a deficiency disease, most children with this diagnosis *are* deficient in certain key nutrients, and do respond very well.

Zinc and magnesium are the most commonly deficient nutrients in people with ADHD. In fact, symptoms of deficiency in these minerals are very similar to the symptoms of ADHD. Low levels of magnesium, for instance, can cause excessive fidgeting, anxious restlessness, insomnia, coordination problems, and learning difficulties (if accompanied by a normal IQ).

Polish researchers studying 116 children with ADHD for their levels of magnesium found that 95 percent of them were deficient in it—a much higher percentage than that among healthy children. The team also noted a correlation between levels of magnesium and severity of symptoms. Supplementing 200 mg of magnesium for six months significantly reduced hyperactivity in the children with ADHD, but behavior in the control group, which received no magnesium, worsened.[13]

Dr. Neil Ward, of the University of Surrey in England, has come up with a finding that could explain the link between ADHD and such deficiencies. In a study of 530 hyperactive children, Ward found that compared to children without ADHD, a significantly higher percentage of children with the condition had been treated several times with antibiotics in early childhood.[14] Further investigations revealed that children who'd had three or more such treatments before the age of three had significantly lower levels of zinc, calcium, chromium, and selenium.[15] This condition probably develops because antibiotics have a disruptive effect on beneficial gut flora and consequently on overall digestive health, as discussed in chapter 9.

Even without supplements, tailoring a child's diet to include higher levels of key nutrients can lead to significant improvements in behavior. Dr. Stephen Schoenthaler of the Department of Social and Criminal Justice at California State University, Stanislaus, has conducted extensive investigations into the relationship between poor diet, nutrient status, and bad behavior.

In his many placebo-controlled studies conducted over eighteen months in Florida and Virginia, which involved over 1,000 long-term juvenile delinquents, Schoenthaler discovered that introducing a better diet improved behavior by 40 to 60 percent. Blood tests for vitamins and minerals showed that around one-third of the young people involved had low levels of one or more vitamins and minerals before the trial, but that by the end of the study, some 70 to 90 percent of those whose levels had risen demonstrated a dramatic improvement in behavior.[16]

Kick Out the Toxic Nasties

Looking beyond low levels of essential nutrients, excess antinutrients can also induce ADHD symptoms. An example of this is copper, which is found in high levels in some children with ADHD. Studies have also revealed a link between high aluminum and hyperactivity. Many toxic elements deplete the body of essential nutrients such as zinc, and may contribute to nutritional deficiencies. A hair mineral analysis to rule out heavy metal toxicity is therefore an important component of an overall nutritional approach. See chapter 7 for more on how to get heavy metals out of your child's system.

THE RISE OF RITALIN

It's a sad fact that many hyperactive children are never evaluated for chemical, nutritional, or allergic factors, nor are they treated nutritionally. Instead, when faced with a child who has ADHD, most doctors immediately write a prescription for a habit-forming amphetamine such as Ritalin, which has many properties similar to those of cocaine. In fact, using brain imaging techniques, Dr. Nora Volkow of the Brookhaven National Laboratory in Upton, New York, has shown that Ritalin is actually more potent than cocaine. So why has prescribing it so widely not produced an army of addicted schoolchildren? Volkow has revealed that it's because it takes about an hour for Ritalin in pill form to affect the brain, while smoked or injected cocaine works in seconds.[17]

Despite these findings, the flood of Ritalin prescriptions shows no sign of abating even though researchers looking at its effectiveness have found that it can worsen the behavior of more children than it helps. Ritalin is now given to up to 20 percent of children in some schools and more than eight million children in the United States are now on the drug—that's a staggering 10 percent of boys aged six to fourteen. Other drugs that are used are slight variations on Ritalin, such as Adderall and Concerta. A newer drug, Strattera (atomoxetine), is also prescribed for ADHD. It works by preventing the reuptake of the neurotransmitter noradrenaline, thus keeping more of it in circulation.

It's thought that the calming effect of drugs like Ritalin and Strattera on hyperactive children is because there is not enough of the neurotransmitter noradrenaline in the part of the brain that is supposed to filter out unimportant stimuli. Dr. Joan Baizer at the University of Buffalo in upstate New York has shown that while Ritalin was previously thought to have only short-term effects, it actually initiates changes in brain structure and function that remain long after the therapeutic effects have dissipated.[18]

Dr. Peter Breggin, a psychiatrist at the International Center for the Study of Psychiatry and Psychology in Ithaca, New York, is an outspoken critic of Ritalin. He says the drug, far from helping children with ADHD, actually damages the brain of the developing child by decreasing blood flow. "Ritalin does not correct biochemical imbalances—it causes them," he says, further alleging that negative research results are being suppressed to protect the enormous profits from the drug's sale.

This assessment of Ritalin is not good news when you consider the U.S. Drug Enforcement Agency's list of side effects from this drug. On top of increased blood pressure, heart rate, respiration, and temperature, people taking Ritalin can experience appetite suppression, stomach pains, weight loss, growth retardation, facial tics, muscle twitching, euphoria, nervousness, irritability, agitation, insomnia, psychotic episodes, violent behavior, paranoid delusions, hallucinations, bizarre behaviors, heart arrhythmias and palpitations, psychological dependence, and even death.[19]

Nor does Ritalin work over time. The National Institutes of Health concluded that there is no evidence of any long-term improvement in scholastic performance on Ritalin.[20] What's more, a child given Ritalin or other stimulant drugs is more likely to become addicted to smoking and abuse other stimulant substances later in life, such as cocaine.[21] The long and short of it is, don't accept a prescription for these drugs on behalf of your child.

Given the possible effect of Ritalin on noradrenaline deficiency in the brain, it is interesting to note that magnesium plays a key role in promoting the production of noradrenaline. And sure enough, the vast majority of children are able to stop taking Ritalin after as little as three weeks once they start supplementing 500 mg of magnesium daily. While giving your child up to 200 mg of magnesium is perfectly safe, we don't recommend larger amounts unless you are under the guidance of a nutritionist. Other nutrients also involved in the production of noradrenaline include manganese, iron, copper, zinc, vitamin C, and vitamin B6, and many of these nutrients are also involved in the proper metabolism of essential fats (see below).[22]

While there is much you can do yourself, ADHD is a complex condition. As such, it really demands supervision and treatment by a qualified practitioner who can devise the correct nutritional strategy for your child. Your child's supplement requirements must be individually assessed, and he will need to follow an optimally healthy diet. A minimum of three to six months may pass before you see any substantial results, but you may well see a general slowing down from hyperactivity and improved concentration in your child very quickly. As your child starts to feel and behave better, the positive feedback he receives from you and his teachers can encourage him to stick to the nutritional program long term—which is what really produces the best results.

REWARD DEFICIENCY SYNDROME

Some children with ADHD also suffer from "reward deficiency syndrome," where they have a constant need for stimulation.[23] This condition is thought to happen because they either don't produce enough of the motivating neurotransmitter dopamine (from which adrenaline and noradrenaline are made), or don't respond strongly enough to their own dopamine.

Drugs like cocaine and Ritalin both increase dopamine production and dopamine sensitivity, at least in the short term. For these children, Ritalin can seem like a miraculous cure. But in the long term, it will cause downregulation so the child will need even more stimulation. This result is probably why children given Ritalin are more likely to abuse other dopamine-promoting drugs and are more likely to become dependent on such drugs later in life.[24]

For these children, the stimulating brain nutrient DMAE (sold as Deanol) is highly effective. Researcher and psychiatrist Dr. Charles Grant discovered that in addition to increasing acetylcholine (the memory neurotransmitter), in higher doses DMAE can actually block the acetylcholine receptor;

this allows more dopamine to be released, thereby stimulating the brain. This action could explain DMAE's proven success with reward deficiency syndrome and ADHD. Unlike Ritalin, DMAE doesn't increase the need for external stimulation and doesn't have all the undesirable side effects.

So, for any child who has ADHD or hyperactivity, we recommend the following steps:

- Follow the guidelines in part 1 regarding nutrients, sugar, essential fats, and heavy metals.
- Eliminate chemical food additives and check other potential allergens such as wheat, dairy, chocolate, oranges, and eggs.
- Consider supplementing DMAE under the guidance of your nutritionist.

Chapter 17

Moving Off the Autistic Spectrum

Few conditions are still as mysterious to us as autism. The autistic spectrum runs all the way from people unable to speak or deal with others, to high-functioning forms such as Asperger's syndrome. The breadth of this spectrum can be startling. For instance, two of the people who have most profoundly shaped our understanding of nature—Einstein and Newton—are now thought by some to have had Asperger's.

All the overlapping conditions in the previous two chapters—dyslexia, dyspraxia, and ADHD—are often present in autism. For this reason, some are beginning to feel that this trio of conditions actually belongs in the autistic spectrum, as the highest-functioning forms. But autism is a distinct condition, with specific symptoms. These include difficulties with speech; abnormalities of posture or gesture; problems with understanding the feelings of others; sensory and visual misperceptions; fears and anxieties; and behavioral abnormalities such as obsessive-compulsive behavior and ritualistic movements. These children also frequently exhibit digestive symptoms such as constipation, diarrhea, and bloating, as well as frequent ear, nose, and throat symptoms. Fits and convulsions are also common in severe autistics—see page 155 for a discussion of the condition and ways to combat it.

Rates of autism have been on the increase for several decades. Some say that this growth is due to increased diagnosis, which may account for some of it. However, while autism used to occur primarily from birth, or at least was detected within the first six months, in both the United States and the United Kingdom over the past ten years there has been a dramatic increase in late-onset autism, most frequently diagnosed at age two; this strongly suggests that something new is triggering an epidemic. Possible culprits include diet, vaccinations, and gastrointestinal problems, which are also very much on the increase in children.

> Six-year-old Andrew is a case in point. He had been diagnosed with autism at age two and a half. He had frequent ear infections and was a very picky eater, often restricting his diet to two foods—chicken nuggets and french fries. Tests revealed that he had a number of food allergies and was low in magnesium. An analysis of his diet showed that he was taking in enormous amounts of sugar. Reducing sugar, supplementing magnesium, and excluding the foods he was allergic to brought about some significant changes. Within a few weeks, his parents noticed and others began commenting that he seemed much brighter and more affectionate and smiled more. He ceased having ear infections and the range of foods that he would eat broadened considerably.

UNRAVELING AUTISM

As with all conditions like this, there is the question as to whether it is inherited or caused by something in diet or environment. Autism is four times as common in boys as girls. Parents and siblings of autistic children are far more likely to suffer from milk or gluten allergy, or have high cholesterol, digestive disorders such as irritable bowel syndrome, night blindness, light sensitivity, thyroid problems, or cancer. Not being breast-fed also increases the risk.

At first glance, it might seem that autistic children inherit certain imbalances. However, an alternative explanation might be that other family members have the same biochemical imbalances, eat the same food, and may be lacking the same nutrients.

Given the overlap with dyslexia, dyspraxia, and ADHD, all the factors discussed in the previous two chapters are also relevant in dealing with autism. So if your child is autistic, you'll need to help her balance blood sugar, check for brain-polluting heavy metals, exclude food additives, identify food allergies, correct digestive problems and possible nutrient deficiencies, and ensure an optimal intake of essential fats. There is growing evidence that these approaches can really make a big difference for children with autism.

Nutrient Deficiencies

We've known since the 1970s that a nutritional approach can help autism, thanks to the pioneering research by Dr. Bernard Rimland of the Autism Research Institute in San Diego. He showed that vitamin B6, C, and magnesium supplements significantly improve symptoms in autistic children. In one of his early studies, in 1978, twelve out of sixteen autistic children improved, then regressed when the vitamins were swapped for placebos.[1] In the decades following Dr. Rimland's study, many other researchers have also reported positive results with this approach.[2]

Still others, however, have failed to confirm positive outcomes with certain nutrients. For example, a French study of sixty autistic children found they improved significantly on a combination of vitamin B6 and magnesium, but not when either nutrient was supplemented alone.[3] This study shows how important it is to get the balance of these nutrients right. It's likely to be different for each child.

B6 in particular may help, in part because many children with autism or learning difficulties have a condition in which, for genetic reasons, high levels of a compound called HPL is excreted in the urine, causing a deficiency of zinc and vitamin B6. All children on the autistic spectrum should be screened for urinary HPL—this involves a simple urine test (see Resources, page 218)—and supplemented with appropriate levels of B6 and zinc.

A Lack of the Right Fats

Deficiencies in essential fats are common in people with autism.[4] Research by Dr. Gordon Bell at Stirling University in Scotland has shown that some autistic children have an enzymatic defect that removes essential fats from brain cell membranes more quickly than it should; this means that an autistic child is likely to need a higher intake of essential fats than average. And it has been found that supplementing EPA, which can slow the activity of the defective enzyme, has clinically improved the behavior, mood, imagination, spontaneous speech, sleep patterns, and focus of autistic children.[5]

The Link with Vitamin A

Pediatrician Mary Megson, from Richmond, Virginia, believes that many autistic children are lacking in vitamin A. Otherwise known as retinol, vitamin A is essential for vision, as we've seen in this book. It is also vital for building healthy cells in the gut and brain. There is no real doubt that something funny is going on in the digestive tracts of autistic children. So how does vitamin A fit into the puzzle?

The best sources of vitamin A are breast milk, organ meats, fish, and cod liver oil, none of which are prevalent in our diets. Instead, we have formula milk, fortified food, and multivitamins, many of which contain altered forms of retinol such as retinyl palmitate, which doesn't work as well as the fish- or animal-derived retinol. Megson began speculating what might happen if these children weren't getting enough natural vitamin A.[6]

She realized that not only would this affect the integrity of the digestive tract, potentially leading to allergies, it would also affect brain development and vision. Both brain differences and visual defects have been detected in autistic children. The visual defects, Megson deduced, were an important clue because lack of vitamin A would mean poor black and white vision, a symptom often seen in the relatives of autistic children.

If you can't see black and white, you can't see shadows. Without shadows, you lose the ability to perceive three-dimensionality; this in turn leaves you less able to make sense of people's expressions, which could explain why some autistic children tend not to look straight at you, but to look at you sideways. Long thought to be a sign of poor socialization, this sideways technique may in fact be the best way for them to see people's expressions, because there are more black and white light receptors at the edge of the visual field than in the middle!

Of course, the proof is in the pudding. And Megson has reported rapid and dramatic improvements in autism simply by giving cod liver oil containing natural, unadulterated vitamin A. Often she has seen results within a week of starting children on the oil.[7] Here are some of the comments her patients have made after cod liver oil supplementation: "Now I know where my fingers are." "Now I can see my arms at the same time I see my fingers!" "Now I can see emotion on the faces on TV."

We recommended cod liver oil supplementation for a seven-year-old with Asperger's. As his mother said, "In the two weeks since following your advice there has been a significant improvement in his eye contact." Although you need to be careful about the overall amounts of this fat-soluble vitamin your child takes (see page 114), vitamin A could be an avenue worth pursuing.

Allergies—Undesirables on Board

In addition to these likely deficiencies, the most significant contributing factor in autism appears to be undesirable foods and chemicals that often reach the brain via the bloodstream because of faulty digestion and absorption. Much of the impetus for recognizing the importance of dietary intervention has come from parents who've noticed vast improvements in their children after changing their diets. As we've seen elsewhere in this book, certain foods and substances appear to adversely influence a large number of children, including:

- Wheat and other gluten-containing grains
- Milk and other dairy products containing casein
- Citrus fruits
- Chocolate
- Artificial food colorings
- Acetaminophen
- Salicylates (see page 137)

The strongest direct evidence of foods linked to autism involves wheat and dairy and the specific proteins they contain—namely, gluten and casein. These are difficult to digest and, especially if introduced too early in life, may result in an allergy. Fragments of these proteins, called peptides, can have big impacts in the brain. They can act directly in the brain by mimicking the body's own natural opioids (such as the enkephalins or endorphins) and so are sometimes called exorphins. Or they can disable the enzymes that would break down these naturally occurring compounds.

In either case, the consequence is an increase in opioid activity, leading to many symptoms we describe as autism. Researchers at the Autism

Research Unit at England's Sunderland University have found increased levels of these peptides in the blood and urine of children with autism.[8]

Gut Feelings

To understand how these common foods can be so harmful to sensitive individuals, we need to look at how they get into the body via the gut.

As we saw above, exorphin peptides are derived from incompletely digested proteins, particularly food containing gluten and casein. One of these, called IAG and derived from gluten in wheat, has been detected in 80 percent of autistic patients.[9] (A urine test for IAG is available from Genova Diagnostics; see Resources, page 218.) So the first problem is the poor digestion of proteins. A lack of sufficient zinc and vitamin B6 could contribute to this, as both are essential for proper stomach acid production and protein digestion yet are often deficient in autistic children with elevated urinary HPL, as we saw above.

Whatever the case, however, partially digested protein fragments shouldn't be entering the bloodstream. So how do they? Vitamin A deficiency is certainly one culprit, but there may be more.

Many parents of autistic children report that their child received repeated or prolonged courses of antibiotic drugs for ear or other respiratory infections during her first year, before the diagnosis of autism. In chapter 9, we saw how broad-spectrum antibiotics kill good as well as bad bacteria in the gut, weakening the intestinal membranes; this can lead to what is known as leaky gut syndrome, in which large molecules that shouldn't be absorbed through the gut membrane do get through.[10] And one kind of these could be exorphin peptides. Recent evidence points to a leaky blood-brain barrier too, meaning more of these exorphins make it to the brain.

When Dr. Andrew Wakefield of London's Royal Free Hospital studied sixty autistic children with gastrointestinal symptoms, he found many more intestinal lesions in them than in nonautistic children with similar digestive problems. In fact, over 90 percent of the autistic children had chronically inflamed guts as a result of infection.[11]

So if your child has autism, restoring a healthy gut is vital. You can start simply by supplementing digestive enzymes and giving probiotics to restore the balance of gut bacteria. Both measures help heal the digestive tract and promote normal absorption and have produced positive clinical results in autistic children.[12] Probiotics may also help your child digest exorphins before they can be absorbed.[13]

The amino acid L-glutamine is also useful for helping to restore the integrity of the digestive tract. It is not suitable for all autistic children, as some appear to have difficulties in processing it, resulting in the production of excess ammonia. Seek the advice of a nutritionist before trying glutamine for your autistic child.

Cutting Out Wheat and Dairy

Adding supplements to your child's diet is important, but so is removing any suspect food. There are many anecdotal reports of dramatic improvements in children with autism from parents who removed casein (milk protein) and gluten (the protein in wheat, barley, rye, and oats) from their diet.[14] It can take some time for harmful peptides to leave the blood and brain, however, so results can be slow to emerge.

Dr. Robert Cade, former professor of medicine and physiology at the University of Florida, observed that as levels of peptides in the blood decrease, the symptoms of autism decrease. "If [levels of peptides] can be reduced to normal range," he writes, "we typically see dramatic improvements." (See figure 17, following page.) But you need to help your child rigidly adhere to a strict gluten- and casein-free diet to accomplish this.[15]

If you decide to go down this route with your child, you'll need to take a slow approach. The Autism Research Unit at Sunderland University recommends a gradual withdrawal of foods, waiting three weeks after the removal of dairy foods (casein) before removing wheat, oats, barley, and rye (gluten) from the diet. Initially, your child may go through "withdrawal" and her symptoms may get worse for a bit.

Keep a food diary and note your child's behaviors and symptoms alongside all the foods she's eating; this can help to identify which of the usual suspects she is sensitive to—citrus fruits, chocolate, artificial food colorings, salicylates, eggs, tomatoes, avocados, eggplant, red peppers, soy, and corn.[16] But remember, most of the foods in this list contain valuable nutrients, too, so you'll have to ensure that they are replaced rather than

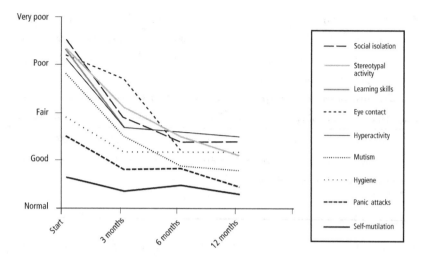

Figure 17. Symptom improvement observed in seventy autistic children while on a gluten- and casein-free diet over twelve months[17]

just removed. As you'll also need to be fully aware of which foods contain gluten and/or casein (see below), this entire process is best done under the guidance of a nutritionist (see Resources, page 217).

Tracking Down Gluten and Casein

Grains containing gluten include wheat (and its close relatives, spelt, triticale, and kamut), oats, barley, and rye. That means you will need to cut out most breads, cookies, cakes, pasta, breakfast cereals, bulgur, couscous, pizza, pita bread, wraps, egg noodles, pastry, bagels, pies, sausages, microwave meals, and processed foods. Check ingredient lists carefully and avoid any products containing flour, malted wheat flakes, modified starch, or wheat starch. Most alternatives are based on rice or corn, and gluten-free breads, pastas, cereals, cookies, crackers, cakes, and bars are now readily available in health food stores and some supermarkets.

Casein is in all dairy products, including cow's milk, butter, cheese, yogurt, ice cream, and milk chocolate. Sometimes goat's or sheep's milk is better tolerated, but you need to remove these from your child's diet too. Make use of the many soy alternatives now available; they include milk, cheese, yogurt, and ice cream. However, soy itself can also be a problem because some people develop sensitivity to it. So don't rely on soy too heavily, and if you suspect your child has developed an intolerance to it, use alternatives made from rice and other gluten-free grains, which are also now widely available in health food stores.

Going for Detox

Peptides can also harm the autistic child via the liver, whose job is that of a sophisticated cleaner's—detoxifying harmful chemicals and breaking down hormones and neurotransmitters.

Through a process called sulfation, the liver inactivates excess amounts of many neurotransmitters that modulate mood and behavior in the brain and so keeps the brain in balance. However, 95 percent of autistic children have low sulfate levels, which may be inadequate for keeping levels of these neurotransmitters in check. Not only that, reduced sulfation also affects the mucin proteins that line the gastrointestinal tract, making the gut leakier and promoting inflammatory bowel disease. And this in turn allows peptides in, where they proceed to reduce sulfate production even further. It's a vicious circle.

The enzyme sulfite oxidase also plays a role in sulfate production, and levels of it are often low in autistic children. Sulfite oxidase is dependent on adequate levels of the mineral molybdenum, so supplementing this can be helpful—about 20 percent of autistic children respond well to it.[18] Also potentially helpful in this context is a highly usable form of sulfur called MSM (methylsuffonylmethane). For advice on dosage, we recommend you consult a nutritionist.

Detoxification of the gut can also be helpful. Autistic children often have dysbiosis, the presence of undesirable microorganisms in the gut, whether bacteria, yeasts, fungi, or parasites. Treatment with antifungal drugs such as Nystatin can get remarkable results, but note that children may get worse before they get better. Other, less aggressive antifungal agents, including charcoal, caprylic acid from coconut, and the yeast *Saccharomyces boulardii*, can be equally effective without triggering really severe reactions.

We strongly recommend you work with a nutritionist, who can advise you and your child on a suitable plan for detoxification, rather than doing it alone (see Resources, page 217, for details).

THE BIG DEBATE—MMR AND AUTISM

Does the MMR (measles, mumps, and rubella) vaccine trigger autism? The issue has been hotly debated in the press and among concerned parents in schoolyards across the United States and beyond. The official line is that there's no good evidence for any link between autism in children and the MMR vaccine. Of course, the last thing the medical profession wants is a whole lot of children not being vaccinated, since that increases the risk of epidemics. But it is true that Dr. Andrew Wakefield's research at the Royal Free Hospital, while important, is only the first hint of a problem, and it is probably too early to jump to conclusions.[19]

It is, however, useful to look at what Wakefield actually said in this context:

> *Although MMR cannot by any means be described as a cause of autism, a child genetically predisposed to asthma, eczema, food allergy or intolerance, perhaps with possible disruption of the gut flora or with a fungal overgrowth, deficient in vitamins, minerals, and essential fats, may be at risk from MMR. For them MMR could be described as the straw that broke the camel's back, tipping the balance of normal childhood development into a retrogressive state.*[20]

For most children, the MMR vaccine is unlikely to be a problem, but that said, no one really knows the full consequences of giving a child three immune attacks—mumps, measles, and rubella—all at the same time. Getting all three illnesses at once simply doesn't occur in nature, so there's a logical argument for single vaccines if a parent so chooses, especially for children with weakened immune systems. Perhaps for children with nutrient deficiencies, a lack of essential fats, and a susceptibility to food allergies, infections, and/or gut problems, these triple vaccines really *are* the last straw.

But is there any hard evidence against the MMR vaccine? First, studies have shown a high incidence of autism in children whose mothers had received live virus vaccines (particularly the MMR or rubella vaccine) immediately before conception or immediately following birth while breast-feeding.[21] Second, there are two classifications of autism: one where autistic traits are noted from birth and one where symptoms are noted at eighteen months plus. The onset of autism at eighteen months was uncommon until the mid-1980s, when the MMR vaccine came into wide use. After that, the incidence shot up.[22]

According to Dr. Bernard Rimland of the Autism Research Institute in San Diego, the problem may not be the vaccine itself, but a preservative used in multidose vials of many childhood vaccines until very recently. Thimerosal, a preservative containing high levels of mercury, was used in many vaccines up until 2001. Before this, each vaccine injection exposed the child to levels of toxic mercury in excess of the U.S. federal government's own safety guidelines, and children receiving all their jabs could have received a total of 187.5 mcg of mercury—enough to give them heavy metal poisoning.[23] However, the removal of thimerosal from all vaccines for young children hasn't been followed by a drop in the incidence of autism.

There's another fact that strengthens the link between autism and the MMR vaccine: many autistic children have been found to have measles antibodies in their gut. It's a bit like having a chronic infection and seems to indicate that the triple vaccine makes measles persist. One of the most important allies the body has to fight off this virus is vitamin A, and Dr. Megson's research (see page 146) indicates that many autistic children lack this key nutrient.

So, although it is too early to say yea or nay conclusively, it is entirely possible that late-onset autism may be triggered by multiple vaccinations, allergies, toxic overload, or nutritional deficiencies, and especially combinations of any of these that send a child's gut and brain into distress.

A NATURAL WAY WITH AUTISM

It can be hard work, but the optimum nutrition approach to helping your autistic child is much more effective than the available drugs and has no negative side effects. It involves healing the digestive tract, avoiding sources of casein and gluten plus any other identified allergens, eating nutritious foods, and supplementing nutrients that help support digestion, absorption, liver detoxification, the immune system, and the brain.

As for drugs such as Ritalin, these are in any case generally not recommended for classic autism, except when it is accompanied by ADHD or hyperactivity. In one survey of 8,700 parents asked to rate the effectiveness of drugs and other interventions, it was found that Ritalin was the most commonly prescribed, but only 26 percent reported any improvement in their child, while 46 percent said their child got worse on it. The most efficient drug in this survey, the antifungal Nystatin, was still found to help only 49 percent of children taking it.[24]

As the story of Habbo clearly shows, the optimum nutrition route can, by contrast, result in tremendous and lasting improvements.

Habbo was diagnosed as autistic at the age of four. He had serious speech and language problems, was severely behind in social and emotional development, and attended special education for children with developmental delay. He had shown some improvement after taking special multivitamins, minerals, and DMG (dimethylglycine, a brain food) prior to visiting a clinic in the Netherlands.

Habbo was given comprehensive biochemical testing for deficiencies and imbalances. The London clinic of the Brain Bio Centre found low levels of five vitamins (A, beta-carotene, B3, B5, and biotin) and three minerals (magnesium, zinc, and selenium). He also had low levels of omega-3 fats and the omega-6 fat GLA, as well as the amino acids taurine and carnitine. His digestion was poor, and he had abnormal gut flora and indications of a yeast infection. Food allergy testing showed a clear sensitivity to milk products and some other foods.

He was given a special diet free from milk and casein, a personalized supplement program, and later the antifungal drug Nystatin. He also started a program of applied behavior analysis, working with a therapist.

He improved steadily and was able to attend his local primary school from the age of six.

According to the Autism Research Institute's evaluation list, his improvements were:

Speech/language	from 36 to 89 percent
Sociability	from 13 to 68 percent
Sensory/cognitive awareness	from 22 to 97 percent
Health/physical behavior	from 64 to 96 percent

(where 100 percent means nonautistic behavior)

By his fifth birthday, Habbo had shown absolutely no interest in presents or visitors. One year after the evaluation, just before his eighth birthday, he made a list of eight presents he would like to have, including a computer. His parents told him the evening before to wake them at 7:30 a.m. on his birthday, and that's exactly what he did. During the day he couldn't wait for his friends to arrive and celebrate his special day.

FITS, CONVULSIONS, AND EPILEPSY

Profoundly autistic children may be prone to epilepsy. Although it's less common, people on the broader autistic spectrum—including ADHD, dyslexia, and dyspraxia—may also have fits or convulsions. Convulsions, which can last for seconds or minutes, are thought to be the result of a temporary upset in the brain's chemistry, causing neurons to fire off faster than usual and in bursts.

Neurological problems such as a brain injury, a stroke, an infection, and, less frequently, a tumor can all bring on convulsions. High levels of stress and panic attacks can also trigger them, as can heart disease, especially irregular heartbeats and blood sugar problems. Whatever the cause, convulsions indicate that the brain is out of balance, so an obvious place to start is to ensure an optimal intake of the brain's best friends—nutrients.

Nutrients That Counter Convulsions

Many researchers have pointed out that people who have convulsions or epilepsy are often deficient in certain nutrients—usually folic acid, the minerals manganese and magnesium, essential fats, and vitamin D.

B VITAMINS

Folic acid is depleted by convulsions, suggesting that it is somehow involved in them.[25] So it is ironic that anticonvulsant drugs such as phenytoin, primidone, and phenobarbital further deplete folic acid.

Combining a drug such as phenytoin with folic acid works better than the drug alone. In one study, epileptics were given this drug with either folic acid or a placebo; after a year, only those on folic acid reported substantially fewer fits.[26] However, folic acid can be a double-edged sword. Some studies without control groups suggest that supplementation with this nutrient may actually cause epileptic fits in a minority of people. Several controlled studies, however, have failed to confirm this observation, suggesting that the incidence must be very rare.[27] With the guidance of your child's doctor, folic acid supplementation is well worth trying, although you can't expect immediate results.

Also worth supplementing is vitamin B6, which in high doses can produce almost immediate results. The first research to identify a role for B6 in the treatment of epilepsy in children took place in Japan in the 1980s. More than half the children with "infantile spasms" responded very well to B6 supplementation, although the doses used were very high and did cause side effects in some participants.[28]

In a more recent study at the University of Heidelberg in Germany, seventeen children were given high doses of vitamin B6 (300 mg/kg per day). Five out of the seventeen had immediate relief within two weeks, while after four weeks all of the patients were more or less free of seizures. No serious adverse reactions were noted. Side effects were mainly gastrointestinal symptoms and were reversible after the dosage was reduced.[29]

MAGNESIUM, MANGANESE, AND ZINC

The mineral manganese is essential for proper brain function, and to date four studies have shown a correlation between low levels of it and epilepsy, with as many as one in three epileptic children having low manganese levels.[30]

In one study, published in the *Journal of the American Medical Association*, one child found to have half the normal blood manganese levels didn't respond to any medication but on supplemented manganese had fewer seizures and improved speech and learning.[31] The late Dr. Carl Pfeiffer, one of the pioneers of nutritional medicine, was the first to report the successful treatment of epilepsy with manganese.[32] At the Brain Bio Centre we have frequently found that patients with convulsions or fits are manganese deficient and have no or fewer fits once supplementation is begun.

Manganese is found mainly in seeds, nuts, grains, and tropical fruit such as bananas and pineapples. (Tea is very rich in it, but we categorically do not recommend children drink tea, as it's a stimulant.)

Magnesium is another mineral well worth checking out if your child is having fits or convulsions. Magnesium is vital for proper nerve and brain function, and once again, a number of researchers have found low levels in patients with epilepsy and reported fewer fits on supplementation.[33] In animals, magnesium injections have also been shown to instantly suppress convulsions.[34]

Of children found to have low blood levels of magnesium, as many as 75 percent respond to supplementation with fewer fits, according to research from Romania.[35] Supplementing this mineral is especially helpful for those with temporal lobe epilepsy, where a person has hallucinations of sound or smell, say, before a fit; this is hopeful news for children with this type of epilepsy, as they rarely respond to conventional anticonvulsant drugs.[36] It is also possible that the children of women who are deficient in manganese while pregnant with them are more likely to be born with epilepsy.

Finally, it's also well worth testing for zinc, as children with epilepsy often have lower levels of this mineral. Ideally, we need to take in ten times more zinc than copper. Zinc is also a valuable ally for vitamin B6, since it helps convert B6 (pyridoxine) into the active form of the vitamin, called pyridoxal-5-phosphate. It is highly likely that the few children who have had adverse reactions to very high doses of vitamin B6 may not have done so if given B6 together with zinc.

In fact, most adverse reactions to vitamins or minerals arise when they are treated like drugs and given at very high doses without other nutrients, thereby completely ignoring the principle of synergy, where nutrients working together amplify each others' actions. For this reason, we strongly recommend that if your child is experiencing fits, convulsions, or epilepsy, you see a nutritional therapist for a thorough nutritional workup, which should involve both hair and blood analyses for magnesium, manganese, and zinc, as well as folic acid. Levels of magnesium and folic acid are best tested in red blood cells. Depending on the results, a nutritional therapist can work out what combination of these nutrients, often in high doses, is worth trying, together with basic multivitamin supplementation.

An all-around good diet and supplements program is, in fact, especially important, since other nutrients have also been shown to have positive effects on mental health in people with epilepsy. These include vitamin B1, selenium, and vitamin E.[37]

VITAMIN D

Vitamin D deficiency may both contribute to seizures and be worsened by epilepsy medication.[38] Vitamin D helps the body to take up calcium, so deficiency in this vitamin can lead to a severe calcium deficiency, a symptom of which is seizures. Several anticonvulsant drugs interfere with the metabolism of vitamin D in the body, which may contribute to or worsen a deficiency. There is a paucity of research in this area, with only one pilot study showing that supplementation of vitamin D reduced seizures.[39] Until more is known, we advise that you have your child's vitamin D levels tested if she has seizures or is on anticonvulsant medication. The best source of vitamin D is sunshine, which may not be sufficiently strong in the northern states during the winter, so if your child has a low level, supplementation may be required. Follow the guidelines in chapter 26 for mild deficiency. For severe deficiency, higher doses may be required under the supervision of a nutritionist or pediatrician.

ESSENTIAL FATS

One of the hottest areas of research into epilepsy is the effect of essential fat deficiency. So many people are deficient in omega-3s, in fact, that it's highly likely a significant proportion of people with epilepsy are also deficient; and there is intriguing evidence to show that supplementation can reduce the incidence of convulsions.

In one study, omega-3 and omega-6 essential fats, in a ratio of 1:4, were given to epileptic rats. After three weeks, up to 84 percent fewer of the rats were having seizures, and the seizures that did occur tended to be very brief—there was up to a 97 percent reduction in their duration. The team of researchers thinks this result was caused by the positive effect of essential fats on stabilizing signals between brain cells.[40]

Omega-3s also work in humans. Researchers at the Kalanit Institute for the Retarded Child in Israel gave children with epilepsy 3 g of omega-3 fats for six months and found a dramatic reduction in both the number and severity of epileptic seizures.[41]

For some years there has been a widely held but unsupported view that omega-6 supplementation may increase the risk of seizures. Fortunately, a recent review of the evidence by Professor Basant Puri of Imperial College, London, has found that the opposite may be true. Omega-6 essential fats are not only safe for epileptics but may also reduce seizure activity.[42]

AMINO ACIDS, PHOSPHOLIPIDS, AND HERBS
Many of the brain food nutrients discussed in part 1, including phosphatidylcholine and essential fats, may also be helpful for children prone to fits. The brain's master tuners—the amino acids SAMe and trimethylglycine (TMG)—are also potential aids (see chapter 14). A close relative of these, dimethylglycine (DMG), produced remarkable results in one twenty-two-year-old man with long-standing learning disabilities, who had been having around seventeen seizures a week despite taking anticonvulsant medication. Within one week of starting 90 mg of DMG twice a day, his seizures dropped to just three a week. When the DMG was withdrawn twice, the frequency of his seizures increased dramatically both times.[43]

The amino acid taurine, which helps to calm down the nervous system, may also help. In animal studies, low concentrations of taurine have been found in parts of the brain where seizure activity is highest, and supplementing taurine was found to have a potent, selective, and long-lasting anticonvulsant effect.[44]

But the real star among these amino acids has got to be GABA, the brain's peacemaker, because it acts directly as a neurotransmitter. One possible mechanism for explaining why anticonvulsant drugs work is that they block the activity of the excitatory neurotransmitter glutamic acid, and thereby promote the inhibitory neurotransmitter GABA.

However, we would be cautious about supplementing GABA, and possibly large amounts of taurine, except under medical supervision, mainly because animal studies have shown that rats prone to petit mal seizures (where they seem absent and stare blankly) sometimes have too much of these amino acids.[45] Another brain-friendly nutrient, the brain stimulator DMAE, while potentially helpful, should also be given with caution. While DMAE is very helpful for many children with attention deficit disorder, a small percentage find it overstimulates, and therefore it should be used with caution—ideally under the guidance of a nutritionist—in children with manic tendencies or a history of epilepsy.

Vinpocetine, an herbal extract derived from the periwinkle plant (*Vinca minor*), may also help with fits, according to research in Russia.[46] This extract does many useful things in the brain, such as improve the production of cellular energy in neurons and widen blood vessels so glucose and oxygen get to the brain more easily and are used more efficiently. As one theory about epileptic fits is that they're caused by fluctuations in glucose or oxygen supplies to the brain, this might explain why vinpocetine works.

So, the message here is that if your child is prone to fits, convulsions, or epilepsy and hasn't been checked out by a nutritionist, there is plenty of room for hope.

If your child has autism, follow the nutritional strategy outlined here along with the recommendations at the end of chapters 15 and 16:

- Eliminate gluten and dairy from your child's diet completely and replace them with the alternatives now readily available, while also checking the possibility of other food sensitivities under the guidance of a nutritional practitioner.

- Give your child cod liver oil, vitamin B6, magnesium, zinc, vitamin C, molybdenum, and high-strength probiotics (minimum four billion micro-organisms) daily.

- Ask your doctor to check your child for urinary HPL, and if she has it, include zinc and vitamin B6 in the above supplement regime.

- When considering the MMR vaccination, if your child has a weak immune system or you suspect nutrient deficiencies, low essential fats, susceptibility to food allergies, infections, and/or gut problems, consider giving her single vaccines if they are available. Alternatively, address all of these issues with a nutritionist prior to your child's receiving the triple vaccine.

If your child has fits, convulsions, or epilepsy, ensure you take the following steps. Note that as the recommended amounts of the supplements listed below depend on the age of your child, it is certainly best to see a nutritional therapist who can work out your child's ideal nutritional strategy.

- Balance your child's blood sugar and check for food allergies.
- Have her vitamin and mineral levels checked. If low in folic acid, B6, magnesium, manganese, zinc, or vitamin D, supplementation may well help.
- Make sure she is getting enough essential fats, from seeds, fish, and their oils.
- Other brain-friendly nutrients and herbs, including amino acids, phosphatidylcholine, DMAE, taurine, and vinpocetine may help, but they are best taken under professional guidance.

Chapter 18

Answers for Aggression

Has your child ever lashed out uncontrollably and violently toward you or someone else? It is a huge shock, and more, it can seem a complete mystery. But be assured that you are not alone. At the Brain Bio Centre, we see many cases of children, some very young, who are uncontrollable and violent. Aggression in children is skyrocketing in the community, too. Sadly, the problem grows with the child, so as difficult as it may be when he is small, as he approaches adulthood his future can look increasingly bleak.

But this scenario is in no way inevitable. You'll already have seen abundantly in this book how today's unbalanced, unhealthful diet affects the brain. And, true to form, we find that the major contributors to aggressive behavior are the usual suspects—too much sugar, not enough essential fats, food allergies, and brain pollution.

Eight-year-old Charles is a case in point. His parents brought him to see us at the Brain Bio Centre because they were concerned about his very aggressive and violent behavior. Tests revealed food allergies, a homocysteine score of 14, and elevated aluminum in his hair. We recommended a specific supplement program designed to reduce homocysteine and to help his body detoxify the aluminum while also avoiding the foods that he was allergic to. After ten weeks, his parents reported that he was much more focused, calmer, and rational and wasn't lashing out like he had been. He had also stopped wetting himself, which had been a problem before.

As we have seen, all thoughts and consequently all behavior are processed through the brain and nervous system, which are—like the rest of the body—completely dependent on nutrition to keep functioning. It's astonishing, but approximately half of all the glucose in the blood goes to power the brain, which is also dependent on a second-by-second supply of micronutrients—vitamins, minerals, and essential fats. Meanwhile, any antinutrients in your child's body, such as lead and cadmium, will fundamentally affect brain function.

To date, there has been very little research into the effects of altering the diet of small children with aggression problems. However, there have been some excellent studies in adolescents, showing dramatic reductions in violent behavior over a short time just by giving them small amounts of essential nutrients. In one study at a juvenile detention center, the teenage inmates were given a multinutrient containing vitamins, minerals, and essential fats, or a placebo. The results of this double-blind trial, published in the *British Journal of Psychiatry*, showed a staggering 35 percent decrease in acts of aggression after only two weeks.[1] Common sense tells us that these nutrients would work even more effectively in small children before these behaviors have become a way of life.

FIGHTING BACK AT AGGRESSIVE BEHAVIOR

We feel there is much you can do to help your child nutritionally if he's often overcome with feelings of anger or engages in aggressive behavior. Let's look at some of the options.

Sorting Out Sugar-Fueled Fury

The involvement of blood sugar fluctuations in behavior is an intimate one. A "rebound low," otherwise known as reactive hypoglycemia, can occur when a child consumes sugar, refined carbs, or stimulants. The rapid rise in blood sugar levels can be followed by a crash, resulting in extreme tiredness, irritability, depression, and aggression. And if a child feels this bad, he's much more likely to behave badly; exhaustion leads to poor impulse control.

If your child's behavior is volatile and out of control, getting to grips with any blood sugar problems is vital. For more on how sugar affects your child's behavior, and what to do to even that out, read chapters 2 and 16.

Omegas—How to Calm Hostility

Recently, deficiency of essential fats has increasingly been seen as a real contributor to aberrant behavior. Changes in modern diets have certainly reduced our intake of these nutrients. And as we've seen, if the mother is deficient during pregnancy, it could have long-lasting effects on the child's mental development and behavior.

Recent research by Dr. Tomohito Hamazaki of Toyama University in Japan suggests that omega-3 fats help control anger and hostility. He reasoned that under conditions of stress a certain level of aggression could have survival value, but from an evolutionary point of view, too much aggression would have the opposite effect.

So he decided to see what would happen to students under the stress of exams if given omega-3 fats. He gave them 1.5 g of DHA or a placebo, measuring hostility using psychological tests at the start of the study and again three months later, just before exams. The second test, just before the exams, showed a 59 percent jump in hostile reactions in those taking the placebo, but no change at all in the students taking the omega-3 fats.[2] Omega-3 fats, it seems, help children to keep their heads under stress.

Countering Nutritional Deficiencies

Essential fats aren't the only key to calmer behavior. Deficiencies in calcium, magnesium, zinc, and selenium have all been shown to correlate with increases in violence.

The simple addition of a multivitamin and mineral supplement containing RDA levels of nutrients has been shown to have extremely positive effects on behavior in prison populations in the United States, according to extensive research by Dr. Stephen Schoenthaler of the Department of Social and Criminal Justice at California State University, Stanislaus, whose work we looked at earlier (see page 138).

In a recent study, Schoenthaler compared the behavior of young offenders in the three months prior to and during supplementation, versus the behavior of those given a placebo. There was an overall reduction in recorded offenses of 40 percent, with the subjects on supplements making 22 percent fewer assaults on staff and reducing violent and nonviolent antisocial behavior by 21 percent compared with the subjects on placebo.

Blood tests for vitamins and minerals showed that around a third of the offenders had low levels of one or more vitamins and minerals before the trial. Those whose levels had become normal by the end of the study demonstrated a massive improvement in behavior of 70 to 90 percent.[3] So it's not rocket science to make the leap that if adequate levels of these nutrients can have such dramatic effects on these adolescents, they will also help younger children with aggressive behavior.

Antisocial Foods

Severe allergic reactions can produce dramatic changes in behavior, as has been well reported in hyperactive children with chemical or food intolerances, as well as in young offenders.[4] Read chapter 9 for more information on brain allergies and how they may lead to seesawing moods.

BIPOLAR CHILDREN

Some children with aggression problems have bipolar disorder, the condition formerly known as manic depression. They may oscillate from states of mania and hyperactivity to crying spells and depression. But the trouble is that bipolar disorder simply isn't diagnosed in childhood. In fact, it used to be thought that it didn't exist in people under twenty, but that is a myth.

Bipolar disorder can and does occur in infancy, but the majority of these children are wrongly classified as having ADHD. Doctors Janet Wozniak and Joseph Biederman from Harvard Medical School found that 94 percent of children with mania also met the criteria for a diagnosis of ADHD. This situation is bad news, because the last thing a child with bipolar disorder needs is stimulant drugs such as Ritalin.

Dr. Demitri Papalos, associate professor of psychiatry at Albert Einstein College of Medicine in New York City, studied the effects of stimulant drugs on seventy-three children diagnosed as bipolar. Disturbingly, he found that forty-seven of these children were thrown into states of mania or psychosis by stimulant medication.[5] His excellent book *The Bipolar Child*, coauthored with his wife, Janice Papalos, helps to differentiate between children suffering from bipolar disorder and children with ADHD.

These are the characteristics and differences they've observed:

- Children with bipolar disorder essentially have a mood disorder and go from extreme highs, with mania, tantrums, and anger, into extreme lows. Some may have four cycles in a year, others weeklong cycles. This rapid cycling is rarely seen in adults.
- Bipolar children also have different kinds of angry outbursts. While most children will calm down in twenty to thirty minutes, bipolar children can rage on for hours, often with destructive, even sadistic, aggressiveness. They can also display disorganized thinking, language, and body positions during an angry outburst.
- Bipolar children have bouts of depression, which is not a usual pattern of ADHD. Many show giftedness, perhaps in verbal or artistic skills, often early in life. Their misbehavior is often more intentional, while the classic ADHD child often misbehaves through being inattentive. A bipolar child can, for example, be the bully in the playground.

The nutritional approach outlined below is likely to be helpful. Ritalin, and other stimulant drugs, can be an absolute disaster.

In summary, we recommend a number of steps for anyone whose child is aggressive or has violent mood swings:

- Remove sugar and additives from your child's diet.
- Check for food allergies.
- See a nutritionist who can test your child for nutrient deficiencies as well as other biochemical imbalances which may be playing a part.
- Aggression is a psychological issue as well as a nutritional one, and you may find you need to follow a complementary approach. Alongside the methods suggested here, consider finding a therapist to address any psychological or family dynamic issues.

Chapter 19

Overcoming
Eating Disorders

A norexia and bulimia are complex and very serious conditions, and they are on the rise. But the good news is that they can be overcome.

If your child has recently become much thinner, how can you know whether she is simply undereating and losing weight or has actually developed an eating disorder? First off, anorexia is very rare in children under twelve, as is bulimia, a condition involving binge eating followed by self-induced vomiting. If your child is under twelve, her thinness could be stemming from allergy, which would make the allergen foods a chore to cope with; or she may have developed a faddy attitude toward certain foods, perhaps egged on by her peers. (For help with food fads, see chapter 22.)

But if your child is twelve or older, it is possible that she is showing anorexic tendencies. She may have been bullied about her weight in school or unconsciously be trying to halt the physical changes of adolescence—and the inexorable progress toward adulthood—by controlling her body shape.

It's important to know what eating disorders look like so you can take appropriate action when and if you need to. See the following chart for signs you need to look out for.

What Is an Eating Disorder?

Physical signs	Behavioral signs	Psychological signs
Anorexia Nervosa		
Severe weight loss No periods (amenorrhea) Hormonal changes in men and boys Difficulty sleeping Dizziness Stomach pains Constipation Poor circulation and feeling cold	Wanting to be left alone Wearing big, baggy clothes Excessive exercising Lying about eating meals Denying there is a problem Difficulty concentrating Wanting to have control	Intense fear of gaining weight Depression Feeling emotional Obsession with dieting Mood swings Distorted perception of body weight and size
Bulimia		
Sore throat or swollen glands Stomach pains Mouth infections Irregular periods Dry or poor skin Difficulty sleeping Sensitive or damaged teeth	Eating large quantities of food Being sick after eating Being secretive	Feeling ashamed, depressed, and guilty Feeling out of control Mood swings
Binge Eating		
Weight gain	Eating large quantities of food Eating inappropriate food Being secretive	Feeling depressed and out of control Mood swings Emotional behavior

Reprinted by permission from **beat** (formerly Eating Disorders Association). Please see www.b-eat.co.uk for more details.

MISSING THE POINT

Anorexia was first identified by Dr. William Gull in 1874. Sufferers eat often vanishingly small amounts of food in an attempt to control out-of-control feelings; they may also exercise obsessively. This was Gull's recommendation for treatment: "The patient should be fed at regular intervals, and surrounded by persons who could have moral control over them, relations and friends being generally the worst attendants."

Today's treatment is unfortunately not much different—summed up as "drug them, feed them and let them get on with their lives" in an article in England's *Guardian* newspaper describing treatment in "leading hospitals." This approach includes behavior therapy using rewards and privileges, and drugs to induce compliance. The drugs include psychotropic drugs such as chlorpromazine, sedatives, and antidepressants. The diet is high-carbohydrate, sometimes as much as 5,000 calories, with little regard for quality.

Bulimia is probably the more common condition nowadays. Some anorexics are also bulimic, but not all bulimics are anorexic. Bulimia involves:

- Recurrent episodes of binge eating (rapid consumption of large amounts of food in a discrete period of time), at least twice a week
- A feeling of lack of control over eating behavior during the binges
- Self-induced vomiting, use of laxatives or diuretics, strict dieting, fasting, or exercise in order to prevent weight gain
- Persistent, obsessive concern with body shape and weight

The underlying reasons for developing such severe and even life-threatening disorders can be numerous and tangled. Many people with anorexia or bulimia bear a secret, a trauma, or a problem that needs to be resolved and can be with the help and support of a psychotherapist.

But there are other possible strands to these difficult and puzzling conditions. Let's look at some of the latest research on nutritional links, which is leading to simple, pragmatic solutions that can work hand in hand with effective therapy.

THE ZINC LINK

The idea that nutrition, or malnutrition, could play a part in the development and treatment of anorexia did not really emerge until the 1970s and 1980s, when scientists began to realize just how similar the symptoms and risk factors of anorexia and zinc deficiency were. As early as 1973, researcher Michael Hambidge concluded that "whenever there is appetite loss in children zinc deficiency should be suspected."[1] In 1979, Rita Bakan, a Canadian health researcher, noticed that the symptoms of anorexia and zinc deficiency were similar in a number of respects, and she proposed that clinical trials be undertaken to test the mineral's effectiveness in treatment.[2]

In fact, many risk factors in the two conditions are identical—both affect women under twenty-five and are linked to stress and puberty, as are many symptoms, including:

- Weight loss
- Loss of appetite
- Amenorrhea (periods stopping)
- Impotence in males
- Nausea
- Skin lesions
- Malabsorption of nutrients
- Disperceptions of self-image
- Depression
- Anxiety

Meanwhile, David Horrobin, most renowned for his research into evening primrose oil, proposed that "anorexia nervosa is due to a combined deficiency of zinc and [essential fats]."[3] More recently, strong evidence has come to light that those with anorexia and bulimia may be more prone to tryptophan deficiency. Tryptophan is the building block for serotonin, the brain's "happy" neurotransmitter, which also helps control appetite.

Confirming the Connection

In 1980, the first trial studying zinc and anorexia started at the University of Kentucky. The researchers discovered that ten out of thirteen patients admitted with anorexia and eight out of fourteen patients with bulimia were zinc deficient on admission. Yet, after ample feeding, they became even more zinc deficient. Since zinc is needed for the digestion and utilization of protein, from which body tissue is made, they recommended that extra zinc, above the amounts that would correct a deficiency, should be given as the anorexic starts to eat and gain weight.[4]

In 1984, the lightbulb went on with two important research findings. The first study, since confirmed, showed that animals deprived of zinc very rapidly developed anorexic behavior and loss of appetite and that if these animals were force-fed a zinc-deficient diet to gain weight, they became seriously ill.[5] The second study showed that zinc deficiency damages the intestinal wall and therefore the absorption of nutrients, including zinc, potentially leading to a vicious spiral of deficiency.[6]

That same year, Professor Derek Bryce-Smith, patron of the Institute for Optimum Nutrition in the UK, reported the first case of anorexia treated with zinc. The patient was a thirteen-year-old girl, tearful and depressed, weighing just 81 pounds. She was referred to a consultant psychiatrist, but despite counseling, three months later her weight was 69 pounds. Then she began a course of zinc supplementation—45 mg a day. Within two months, she weighed 98 pounds and was cheerful again, and tested normal for zinc levels.[7]

In the mid-1980s, meanwhile, the first double-blind trial with fifteen anorexics began at the Department of Pediatrics at Stanford University Medical Center. In 1987 the researchers reported, "Zinc supplementation was followed by a decrease in depression and anxiety. Our data suggest that individuals with anorexia nervosa may be at risk for zinc deficiency and may respond favorably after zinc supplementation."[8] By 1990, many researchers had found that over half of anorexic patients showed clear biochemical evidence of zinc deficiency.[9]

Zinc supplementation couldn't be easier, but sadly many treatment centers still fail to offer it.

Chicken or Egg?

The evidence linking zinc and anorexia is now beyond question. In fact, a recent review of all the research so far concludes, "There is evidence that suggests zinc deficiency may be intimately involved with anorexia in humans: if not as an initiating cause, then as an accelerating or exacerbating factor that may deepen the pathology of anorexia."[10]

But the fact that high levels of zinc supplementation help to treat anorexia does not mean that the cause of anorexia is zinc deficiency. It is psychological issues that usually trigger changes in the eating habits of susceptible people.

As mentioned above, anorexia can be a way of staving off adulthood and what are perceived as overwhelming fears and responsibilities. By avoiding eating, a young girl can repress the signs of growing up. Menstruation stops, breast size decreases, and the body stays small. Starvation also induces a kind of high by stimulating changes in important brain chemicals that may help to block out difficult feelings and issues that are too hard to face.

So where does zinc come in? Many anorexics choose to become vegetarian, and most vegetarian diets are lower in zinc, essential fats, and protein, according to a study at the Health Sciences Department of the British Columbia Institute of Technology in Burnaby, Canada, which analyzed the diets of vegetarian anorexics versus nonvegetarian patients.[11]

Whether vegetarian or not, once the pattern of not eating is chosen and becomes established, zinc deficiency is almost inevitable, due to both poor intake and poor absorption. With it come a further loss of appetite and even more depression and impaired perception, along with an inability to cope with the stresses that face many adolescents growing up in the twenty-first century.

The optimum nutrition approach to helping someone with anorexia or bulimia is best adopted alongside sessions with a skilled psychotherapist. The nutritional approach emphasizes quality of food rather than quantity, including supplements to ensure vitamin and mineral sufficiency, including 45 mg of elemental zinc a day, and half that once weight gain is achieved and maintained.

TRYPTOPHAN AND APPETITE

A loss of weight and of muscle tissue indicates protein deficiency. Obviously, with anorexia or bulimia, the sufferer will not be getting enough protein, or she may be having trouble digesting, absorbing, or metabolizing it. The amino acids valine, isoleucine, and tryptophan have been found to be low in people with anorexia. Supplementing valine and isoleucine helps to build muscle, while tryptophan is the building block of serotonin, which controls both mood and appetite.

Recent research has found striking differences in the level of tryptophan in the blood of people with anorexia.[12] Both starvation and excessive exercise have emerged as factors in these levels.[13] So far, the evidence points to problems with how anorexics or bulimics respond to low levels of tryptophan. As the conversion of tryptophan into serotonin is both zinc and B6 dependent, all three nutrients may be needed for proper appetite control, as well as a balanced, happy mood.

The interplay between body and mind, or nutrients and behavior, is well illustrated by recent research at Oxford University's psychiatry department by Dr. Philip Cowen and colleagues. Cowen and his team found, not surprisingly, that levels of tryptophan and serotonin were lower in women on calorie-restricted diets. They also found, however, that recovered bulimics put on a diet free of tryptophan rapidly became more depressed and overly concerned about their weight and shape, as well as more fearful of losing control over their eating.[14]

Looked at together, all this research strongly suggests that people prone to anorexia or bulimia have a special need for tryptophan, and probably zinc and B6, and that when deprived of these nutrients they are more likely to develop unhealthy responses to stress, such as the loss of appetite control.

The most direct way of addressing these imbalances in people with eating disorders is to supplement tryptophan, or 5-hydroxytryptophan (5-HTP), plus zinc and B6. But in the long run, the goal has got to be a change in diet. Often, especially in anorexics, supplements such as concentrated fish oils are easier to handle at the start because, unlike food, they contain virtually no calories. As the person's nutritional status improves, her anxieties and obsessive-compulsive tendencies will ease off, and she will almost always see the logic of making positive dietary changes.

The ideal diet should include foods that are easy to eat and digest, as well as highly nutritious. Good-quality protein such as quinoa, fish, soy, and spirulina or blue-green algae is important, as are ground seeds, lentils, beans, fruits, and vegetables.

Fish and seeds are especially important because they contain essential fats. Since most people with eating disorders go out of their way to avoid fat, their diets are frequently low in these essential nutrients, which as we've seen really are essential when it comes to mental health. Also, essential fats are vital for both making serotonin and receiving the serotonin signals that cross from one neuron to another, spreading the happiness around, in effect.

PINNING DOWN BINGE FOODS

The foods people with bulimia binge on are highly revealing, either of food sensitivities or blood sugar problems. The most common binge foods are sweet, wheat-based, or dairy products. Both wheat and dairy products contain exorphins, chemicals that mimic (and can therefore block) pleasure-giving endorphins in the brain, and so possibly influence behavior. And when the person's blood sugar is very low—as it would be after a fast or after vomiting—they would inevitably crave sweet foods for a quick sugar fix.

The effects of all these foods can contribute to the confusion and erratic or compulsive behavior of people struggling with bulimia. We often ask people with bulimia to binge as much as they like for the next two weeks, but not on any of these foods. Many of them report that their desire to binge at all is dramatically reduced right away.

Don't think, however, that if your child is, say, more prone to react strongly to the lack of a nutrient like zinc or tryptophan, that that's the whole story. As we have said, biochemistry does not exclude psychological problems as part of the reason your child has developed an eating disorder. Seek constructive help from a sensitive and reliable therapist.

We have the following recommendations for anyone who is dealing with an eating disorder:

- See a nutritionist who can assess what your child is deficient in and advise you accordingly.
- The nutritionist's recommendations will probably include zinc, B6, and 5-HTP, plus essential fats, either in capsules or in seeds and fish.
- Take your child to see a therapist with experience helping children with eating disorders make a full recovery.

Chapter 20

Curing Sleep Problems

C an't sleep, won't sleep? Children's sleep problems are some of the most common parents face. The result isn't just mentally exhausted children who struggle to learn, concentrate, and behave, but also parents in a permanent state of tiredness themselves. Research showed many years ago that one key to growth and development in children is a good night's sleep, and that includes the growth and development of the brain.

So poor sleep delivers a double whammy: a short-term impact on your child's performance, energy, and mood today, and an insidious curb on his development that prevents him from reaching his full potential as an older child and adult.

Seven-year-old James is a case in point. His mother brought him to see us at the Brain Bio Centre because, no matter how tired he became, he simply was not sleeping. Consequently, he had terrible concentration and memory in school. We screened him for various biochemical imbalances and analyzed his diet. We found that James had food allergies, low levels of calcium and magnesium, and too much sugar in his diet. By excluding the foods that James was allergic to, reducing his sugar intake, and supplementing extra calcium and magnesium, James's sleep improved significantly within a matter of weeks.

IS YOUR CHILD SLEEP DEPRIVED?

Without sleep, even for a night, the body shows clear signs of stress: mood and concentration go, defenses drop, zinc and magnesium levels fall, and vitamin C is used up at an alarming rate. Sleep rejuvenates both body and mind. In fact, during the first three hours of sleep, the body goes into rapid repair mode.

Sleep specialists at Loughborough University in the UK have carried out a series of tests into how the brain functions when it is deprived of sleep. And the results are very clear: sleepy people have problems finding the right words, coming up with ideas, and coping with rapidly changing situations.[1] Sleep deprivation makes us moody and irritable and, in the long term, even depressed. Scientists have measured the body's ability to fight off infections when it is tired, and research has shown that sleep-deprived individuals have fewer natural killer cells, a type of immune cell needed for resistance against invaders.[2]

School-aged children need somewhere from nine to twelve hours of sleep at night. It's easy to tell if they're getting enough: they go to bed, fall asleep easily, wake up easily, and are never tired during the day.

There are two main types of sleep problems—trouble getting to sleep and trouble staying asleep. If your child resists going to bed and kicks up a fuss every night at bedtime, it could be that he faces the inevitable prospect of lying awake for hours feeling bored and frustrated before he finally drops off. And a television, video game console, or computer in the bedroom is not the answer, since research shows that these make sleep problems worse.

Judith Owens of Brown University School of Medicine studied 495 children in kindergarten and primary school to determine what effect watching TV might have on their sleep patterns. She found that TV watching at bedtime, especially when the set was in the child's bedroom, was the strongest predictor of a bad night's sleep, with the child taking longer to get to sleep and being more likely to wake in the night.[3]

A recent report links cell phone use with sleep problems. People using a cell phone before bed take longer to reach deep sleep states and spend less time in them, which gives the body less time to repair itself.[4]

If your child is struggling to sleep, make his bedroom an electronics-free zone!

FINDING THE ZZZZZ FACTOR

Whichever type of sleep problem is affecting your child, the factors to consider are the same: along with habitual television watching last thing at night, these include deficiencies of the calming minerals magnesium and calcium, excess sugar or stimulants, food allergies, and a lack of physical activity during the day.

Chill-Out Minerals

If your child fails to get enough magnesium and calcium, it can trigger or exacerbate sleep difficulties because these minerals work together to calm the body and help relax nerves and muscles. As we've seen, magnesium deficiency is increasingly common in children.

In fact, your child's diet is likely to be lower in magnesium than in calcium, so make sure he's eating plenty of magnesium-rich foods—seeds, nuts, green vegetables, whole grains, and seafood. Including some magnesium in the evening, perhaps even in a supplement, may help. If a breast-fed baby is having trouble sleeping, the mother can take a magnesium supplement and her baby will receive it through her milk. Particularly good sources of calcium, meanwhile, include milk products, green vegetables, nuts, seafood, and molasses.

Other nutrients that are important for good sleep are the B vitamins. These are best taken earlier in the day rather than in the evening, though, as they are also involved in energy production and can be overstimulating just before bed.

Cutting Out Stress, Sugar, and Stimulants

Many of the daily rhythms in your child's body, including those dictating energy and sleepiness, are finely tuned mechanisms that depend on certain hormonal patterns, chemicals, and nutrients. At night, his levels of the stress hormone cortisol should dip, calming him down and preparing his body for sleep. If, however, his cortisol levels are out of balance for any reason (usually stress or a diet high in stimulants or sugar), his ability to get to sleep, to sleep through the night, or to wake up refreshed are likely to be impaired.

If cortisol levels are high at night, for instance, this suppresses the release of growth hormone, which is essential for daily tissue repair and growth. So it's an excellent idea to establish a twenty- to thirty-minute nightly calm-down bedtime routine, which can include taking a bath, putting on pajamas, reading, and other relaxing activities.

Many parents whose children wake in the night and then can't get back to sleep find that keeping their child's blood sugar levels even during the day sets the scene for the correct patterns at night, giving them more chance of a good night's sleep. A light, low-GL snack half an hour to an hour before bed ensures not only that your child is not kept awake by hunger pangs, but also that he won't be woken during the night by a drop in blood sugar levels. A small piece of fruit and a handful of seeds, or some nut butter on one or two oatcake crackers is ideal. Caffeine—and this includes chocolate—should be avoided entirely. Even small amounts taken early in the day can keep children awake at night.

Solving Sleep Apnea

Children who have a chronically blocked nose may suffer from sleep apnea, a condition usually associated with older adults. In sleep apnea, your sleeping child will struggle to breathe to the point of waking up, or at least will have a very restless night. If your child has a stuffy or runny nose and is a mouth breather, you should suspect food allergies.

Read chapter 9 for details on identifying and eradicating food allergies. Addressing food allergies can also be the answer for other sleep-associated problems such as bed-wetting.

Serotonin and Melatonin

The amounts of serotonin and the hormone melatonin in our bodies increase in the evening as part of our natural sleep-wake cycle. Deficiencies in either can prevent sleep, and disruptions in sleep patterns can deplete the body of these substances. The body needs adequate amounts of B6 and tryptophan to make serotonin and melatonin.

Foods particularly high in tryptophan are chicken, cheese, tuna, tofu, eggs, nuts, seeds, and milk. So, as so often happens, a traditional remedy—

drinking a glass of milk before bed—has become grounded in science. (Other foods associated with inducing sleep are lettuce, which contains a substance related to opium, and oats.)

The amino acid our bodies use to make serotonin and melatonin is 5-HTP, so supplementing 5-HTP for a month can be useful as a way of normalizing sleep patterns, once all the other obstacles to sleep have been addressed. When your child is sleeping well again, he can stop taking the supplements. We recommend 25 g an hour before bed for children under eight, and 50 mg for older children.

Melatonin production in the body is lowered by bright light, so make sure all the lights in your child's bedroom are dimmed before he goes to sleep. You can get up to 50 mcg of melatonin in a 3-ounce (85 g) serving of oats, brown rice, or corn. Bananas and tomatoes have half this amount. So serving these foods in the evening may help your child sleep.

Melatonin is a neurotransmitter, not a nutrient, and hence needs to be used much more cautiously when supplementing. Taking too much can cause diarrhea, constipation, nausea, dizziness, headaches, depression, and nightmares. However, melatonin has been used to good effect in children in a number of studies, so is worth a try under the guidance of a nutritionist.[5]

Running Out the Restlessness

Have you ever watched your child running around a playground and thought, "He'll sleep well tonight"? It's true: exercise releases stress and promotes calmness and a sense of well-being, partly through the release of endorphins. So aside from exercise class in school, encourage your child to get active on weekends and in the afternoon rather than simply slumping in front of the TV or computer. He's sure to find something he enjoys: swimming, football with friends, tennis, dance class, or just a brisk walk in the park or a spin on his bike. Just ensure he doesn't exercise too late in the evening, as the energizing effects of all that activity may promote sleeplessness.

To ensure your child get a good night's sleep, follow these sensible suggestions:

- Avoid sugar and stimulants, especially after 4:00 p.m.
- Follow a regular, calming bedtime routine every evening.
- Supplement magnesium and calcium in the evening and ensure your child eats plenty of magnesium and calcium-rich foods such as seeds and crunchy or dark green vegetables.
- To reestablish a good sleep pattern, try 10 to 25 mg of 5-HTP, and perhaps melatonin under supervision.
- Limit television to no more than two hours a day, and if there is a television, computer, or video game console in your child's bedroom, remove it.
- Ensure your child has plenty of stimulating physical activity during the day so he is ready for sleep in the evening.

PART 4

Food for Thought

Now that you know what optimum nutrition for your child's mind really means, how do you put this into action? In this part of the book, we'll show you what to do to feed your child properly, from infancy to teenage years. You'll find shopping tips, meal ideas, and practical ways to keep your child's diet on track and to choose the right supplements.

Chapter 21

Getting Off to
a Good Start

Ideally, optimum nutrition for your child starts with you. If you're optimally nourished before you even conceive, and all the way through pregnancy and breast-feeding, you're giving your child a brilliant head start in life.

Breast milk is, in fact, your child's optimum food for robust physical and mental health during those crucial first few months. Developing good food habits starts with the weaning process, when your two main objectives need to be keeping your child from developing food allergies and ensuring she develops a taste for a wide range of healthy foods.

THE SMART WAY TO FEED YOUR BABY

As a way of nourishing your baby, breast-feeding is better by design. And not just for her physical development: breast-fed babies are not only healthier all around and less prone to obesity and allergies in later life,[1] they are also smarter! A recent analysis of studies concluded that breast-fed babies have "significantly higher scores for cognitive development" than formula-fed babies.[2]

One reason for this is probably the high levels of the omega-3 fat DHA that are found naturally in breast milk. As we've seen, DHA is vital for brain development. And the longer a baby is breast-fed, the higher the intelligence she can expect to have as a young adult.[3] Another reason for the higher intelligence is likely to be that the fat-soluble vitamins in breast milk are more easily absorbed.

In a Brazilian study, only 1 in 176 breast-fed babies had lower than adequate levels of vitamin E, compared to more than half in a cow's milk formula–fed group.[4] There are also more brain-boosting minerals in breast milk than in most formulas.[5]

Breast-feeding also helps to establish healthy gut bacteria. A type of beneficial gut bacteria called bifidobacteria, present in breast milk but not formula milk, prevents harmful bacteria from invading your baby's gut. This is an important service, as it not only protects against colic, eczema, and asthma, but crucially, as we saw in chapter 9, also helps to prevent food allergies, which can affect the brain.

Breast-fed babies are also less likely to be obese. A study of 32,000 Scottish children three to four years old found that those breast-fed for six to eight weeks after birth were 30 percent less likely to be obese than bottle-fed children.[6] As the quality of your milk while breast-feeding is determined to a large extent by the quality of your diet, you'll need to be optimally nourished yourself and also avoid any foods you might be allergic to since you can pass on food allergies through breast milk. (For more information on healthy nutrition during pregnancy and breast-feeding, read *Optimum Nutrition Before, During, and After Pregnancy,* by Patrick Holford and Susannah Lawson.)

KEEPING YOUR CHILD ALLERGY FREE

As with so much else, prevention is better than cure when it comes to allergies and your child. Preventing an allergy from developing in your child is much easier and better than trying to cure her later. There are two important points here: one is the choice and timing of first foods, the other the health of your baby's digestive system.

First Foods

Don't start weaning your child onto food earlier than you need to—start at around six months. It's preferable to breast-feed your baby exclusively up to this point. If she is failing to thrive on breast milk alone, visit your pediatrician or nutritionist for advice before deciding to add other foods to her diet. A lack of solid foods or formula milk may not be the problem, and adding these to her diet may make things worse if poor digestion is an issue.

Since, as we saw in chapter 9, some foods are more likely to cause aller-gies than others, a strategic introduction of the least allergenic foods into your baby's diet while her digestive tract is still immature is essential.

What and When to Introduce While Weaning

From 6 months

- Vegetables *except* tomatoes, potatoes, bell peppers, and eggplant (members of the nightshade family)
- Fruits *except* citrus
- Legumes and beans
- Rice, quinoa, millet, and buckwheat
- Fish (preferably organic, wild, or deep-sea)

From 9 months

- Meat and poultry (preferably organic)
- Oats, corn, barley, and rye
- Live yogurt
- Tomatoes, potatoes, bell peppers, and eggplant
- Eggs
- Soy (as in tofu or soy milk)

From 12 months

- Citrus fruits
- Wheat
- Dairy products
- Nuts and seeds

It's a good idea to start a weaning diary so you can keep track of how your baby takes to the various foods you introduce. To begin with, intro-duce only one food each day, make a note of it, and watch for any possible reaction. A reaction could be anything from a skin rash or eczema, exces-sive sleepiness, a runny nose, or an ear infection, to dark circles under the eyes, excessive thirst, overactivity, or asthmatic breathing. If you notice anything amiss, stop giving that food and then introduce another once the

reaction has died down. You can double-check your observations by rein-
troducing these foods a few months later. By that time, your baby's digestive system will have matured, so she may no longer react to that food.

Once your baby is eating a mixture of foods that cause no reaction, it's
then important to vary her diet as much as possible, especially with common allergenic culprits such as wheat, dairy, soy, and citrus fruits. Eating
the same thing over and over again long term can overtax the system and
induce an allergy. A varied diet will also boost your child's desire for a
wider range of foods, and this will in turn ensure she's getting a broader
range of nutrients.

Digestive Health

Food allergies are intimately linked to poor digestive health—one seems
to exacerbate the other. But keeping your baby's gut healthy is vital for a
lot of other reasons, too.

For instance, the gut and brain are closely connected via the nervous
system, so closely that the gut is actually thought of as a second brain.
Called the enteric nervous system, this network of neurons, neurotransmitters, and proteins lining the gut is in constant communication with the
central nervous system up in your brain and spinal cord. So keeping your
child's gut healthy is also essential for optimizing her brain development.

Unfortunately, many babies these days seem to have their first dose of
antibiotics within days or weeks of birth, resulting in gastric upsets and
more. Antibiotics wipe out the beneficial gut flora in the digestive tract,
causing an imbalance in them that can in turn lead to food allergies, digestive problems, and lower levels of essential minerals.[7] Links have even been
found to ADHD.[8]

Antibiotics are usually given to babies for ear, nose, and throat infections, which may themselves be caused by food allergies, particularly if
they are recurrent. So it is well worth getting to the root of the problem
and resolving food allergies. According to a study published in the *Journal
of the American Medical Association*, antibiotics given for ear infections in
children triples the chance of a repeat infection![9]

While breast milk contains beneficial gut flora that will recolonize your
baby's gut following antibiotics, formula milk typically doesn't. If it's essential for your baby to take antibiotics, make sure you follow them with an

age-appropriate probiotic supplement that will supply the right strains of gut flora.

A GOOD DIET FROM THE START

Once your child is onto solids, the next eighteen months are absolutely crucial to establishing nutritious eating. The emphasis should be on vitamin- and mineral-rich vegetables and fruit. Choose organic if you can, so you are not polluting your baby with residues from artificial fertilizers, herbicides, or pesticides.

Many parents make the mistake of weaning their child onto a lot of fruit and "baby cereals," both of which are very sweet. If you do this, you may find your child rejecting vegetables. So really prioritize vegetables over fruit. The less sweet food and drink your baby has, the less she will desire it. Also, remember that while you are spoon-feeding mashed carrot into your baby's mouth, she's watching your facial expression. So look like you enjoy eating it too! It's very easy to unconsciously let your face screw up into a grimace while cooing "Mmmm yummm" to your baby. She won't be fooled if your *face* is saying "Ooh yuck!"

Make sure, too, that there's plenty of colorful variety. Dr. Gillian Harris, a clinical psychologist at Birmingham University in the UK, has studied the impact of first foods on a child's food preferences later on. She found that babies weaned on baby food, processed foods, and milk are more likely to go on to prefer "beige carbohydrates" such as white bread and chips rather than eating their greens. Babies exposed to fruit, vegetables, and a range of other colorful foods will, by contrast, show a greater preference for many-hued, nutrient-laden foods later on.

Dr. Harris attributes this to an ancient survival mechanism. She believes that children build up a "visual prototype" of favored foods. This model meshes with evolutionary theory, which suggests that our tastes and preferences were shaped to help us survive.

We are born with a love of sweet tastes, associated with ripe fruit and breast milk, and a dislike of bitter tastes, linked for obvious survival reasons with alkaloid toxins in plants. But we can learn to change these tastes depending on what our parents give us to eat. However, at the age of around eighteen months, when a Stone Age toddler would have been able to wander around and select her own food for the first time, the visual prototype mechanism is turned on to prevent her from wanting to eat unfamiliar and potentially poisonous foods.

DOES MY CHILD NEED TO DRINK MILK?

For as long as you breast-feed, you don't need to supplement your baby's diet with cow's milk. However, once you stop, you will need to ensure she gets a good source of calcium. Milk has been marketed for decades as the perfect calcium-rich food, especially for young children. But the key word here is "marketed."

Early humans drank no milk after weaning—yet they still managed to develop strong bones and teeth. There is no evidence that once they ceased to be nomadic hunter-gatherers and began to cultivate the land, eating grains and keeping animals for meat and milk, their bones got stronger. In fact, the opposite seems to be true. We appear to have shrunk in height by five or six inches! This outcome, however, is thought to be due to difficulties in dealing with grain, more than to any problem with milk.[10]

We need to remember that milk is a specialized food full of hormones geared for calves, rather than us. And as we've seen, milk protein or casein causes digestive problems in a lot of people. Meanwhile, if it is so essential, where do the Chinese (for instance), whose consumption of milk is vanishingly small, get their calcium? From vegetables, nuts, seeds, and soy products. So while it's widely consumed by our society, milk doesn't seem to stand up as an essential for good health. And since many people develop allergies to it, it's not a good idea for your child to become too reliant on milk—as long as you make sure her diet is rich in other sources of calcium. See the following table for the best calcium-rich foods, which are important inclusions in your child's diet if you're restricting dairy products.

If you decide you do want to give your child milk, reduce its allergic potential by rotating cow's milk with goat's and sheep's milks, plus soy, rice, and nut milks (although you need to wait until she is a year old before introducing any nut products). Visit your local health food store to find a full selection. We ourselves buy a variety and switch between them, using up one carton before starting on a different type of milk.

Yogurt is often better tolerated than milk, as the live bacteria that make it predigest a lot of the problematic milk sugars and proteins. Live yogurt, especially, where these bacteria remain intact, can help to promote a healthy digestive system. And the calcium in yogurt is easier to absorb than that in milk. Goat's and sheep's yogurt is easy to find these days, allowing you more variety.

Calcium in Foods—The Richest Sources

Per 100 g/100ml	Calcium content (mg)
Cheddar cheese	720
Tahini (sesame seed paste)	680
Sesame seeds	670
Sardines canned in oil	550
Almonds	240
Spring greens, raw	210
Watercress	170
Brazil nuts	170
Kale	150
Tofu (enriched with calcium)	150
Blackstrap molasses (per tablespoon)	150
Whole milk	115

To get your child off to the best start in life, follow these rules:

- Breast-feed exclusively for about six months, then wean her following the guidelines in this chapter.
- During weaning, introduce plenty of colorful vegetables rather than bland, sweet fruit or cereal mixes. And as you demonstrate eating it to your baby, look like you're enjoying it too!
- If your baby is given antibiotics, follow them with age-appropriate probiotics to replenish the beneficial gut flora. Seek advice from a nutritionist.

Chapter 22

Preventing Food Fads and Fussiness

I
f your baby is a fussy eater, he's setting the scene for a lifetime of fussy eating. So it's up to you to do something about mealtime pickiness. It may simply seem an annoyance, but the truth is that by turning up his nose at a variety of food, your child is missing out on the rich range of brain-boosting nutrients we've covered in this book.

You need to start early to ensure that your child actively enjoys eating a broad variety of nutritious foods. If you leave it until he's older, the refusals will become more and more ingrained, and your child will in any case listen to you less and less as he approaches his teen years!

"MY CHILD WILL ONLY EAT . . ."

Which is it? Chocolate yogurt? Pancakes with maple syrup? Fries? Potatoes, carrots, and sausages? If you haven't said, "My child will only eat . . . ," you'll have heard it in the schoolyard or on the phone from a desperate fellow parent. If you have missed the window of opportunity in your child's infancy to nip his fussy-eating tendencies in the bud (see chapter 21), all is not lost—but now is the time to act.

First, go through your cupboards and fridge. If you don't actually store sugary yogurts, soda, chips, or whatever other junk food your child says he wants to eat, you have the perfect answer to his request: there isn't any. Meanwhile, you can be stocking up on wholesome alternatives to the foods he likes.

For homemade chocolate yogurt, you could add carob powder to live yogurt. Instead of pancakes with maple syrup, you could make savory pancakes with whole wheat flour, served with an egg. In place of garishly colored sodas, give him orange juice mixed with sparkling water. But make the changes gradually. Be patient, persistent, and as sneaky as you have to be. For instance, if your kid has always balked at eating vegetables, you can add peas and sautéed, pureed zucchini to pasta sauce or make vegetable soups that you put through the blender. (For detailed tips on making nutritious changes in the kitchen, see chapter 24.)

As ever, your own attitude to food is vitally important. If you're not keen on eating your greens, it's no surprise when your children follow suit! Notice your tone of voice when you offer different foods. You'll probably find that you present foods you yourself really like in an excited way. If carrots and broccoli don't sing to you, *you* need to get excited about vegetables too, and that might mean learning new ways to prepare them. Buy some new cookbooks that focus on fresh, wholesome ingredients.

Ultimately, you'll need to eat well if you want your children to eat well. So the quest to optimally nourish your child will by necessity draw you into this way of eating, too, which can hardly be a bad thing!

NO BRIBES, REWARDS, OR PUNISHMENTS

Taking the emotion out of mealtimes can also help if you have a fussy eater. The majority of food fads are emotionally driven—often vehicles for your child to get attention or assert his independence. So the fewer emotions you display at the breakfast or dinner table, the better. For example, try not to praise your child lavishly for emptying his plate and don't appear too hurt when your lovingly prepared vegetable casserole goes uneaten. Also, don't bribe or reward your child with sweet foods, punish him for not eating, or force him to eat.

From the very start, eating should be a matter of satisfying appetite, not something done for Mommy (or even for starving people). Nor does it need to be a tidy activity. So let your child's appetite, not your desire to feed him, be the governing factor at mealtimes. If he wants more food one day, give it to him—he could be preparing for a growth spurt. Equally, if his hunger wanes the next day, don't force-feed him. He may be unwell or just tired.

Eating should also be an independent activity. As soon as your child can use a spoon or his hands—whichever is easier and (for his enjoyment) messier—encourage him to do so. So don't be too tough too soon on your child's manners. Let him learn to enjoy food first and eat it tidily later.

MANAGE YOUR CHILD'S CHOICES

If your child is very young, it will be a few years before he can knowledgeably make a choice between, say, risotto or pasta. As a toddler, he will not understand if you ask, "What do you want for lunch today?" He may respond if you hold up a banana and a pear and ask, "Do you want a banana or a pear?" And with an older child, it's better to give him a choice of two or three foods rather than asking the open question "What would you like to eat?"

Research shows that children are more willing to eat the food they themselves have chosen. So while you need to keep this simple to avoid overwhelming your child or even encouraging fussiness, you can involve him more as he grows. For example, ask him to pick out some fruit and vegetables in the supermarket, or get him involved in preparing meals. Cooking for optimum nutrition is not only fun, it will also set him up for a lifetime of nutritious eating and give him a real alternative to the ubiquitous junk food that so many teenagers succumb to.

KEEP SNACKS SIMPLE

Snacks are important for keeping blood sugar even and energy stores topped up, but having too many may prevent your child from eating proper meals. If it looks as if this is happening, don't give interesting foods as snacks. If your child is really hungry between meals, he will happily eat a carrot stick or an apple—so keep plenty of these in the fridge, and supply a sealed plastic box with raw vegetables or a bit of fruit for schooldays too.

Note that drinking lots of milk can also dampen appetite, as it's a food and quite filling. If you notice your child is guzzling milk between meals, remind him that there's water or diluted fruit juice to drink, too.

Be careful too, of rewarding or comforting your child with frequent snacks—this can lay down emotional patterns that may later encourage him to eat for comfort when faced with a difficult situation, which, in the long term, can lead to obesity. Three meals and two snacks a day, with raw vegetables freely available, should keep him going.

EATING OUT

While you can provide your child with wholesome food at home, keeping this up can be difficult when he visits friends or goes to parties, or when your family eats out or goes on vacation. But as long as his basic diet is the best it can be, the occasional bag of chips or bowl of chocolate ice cream is fine. And if you explain that there's one way of eating at home and another way elsewhere, you can help your child associate these "treats" with special occasions and not pester you for them all the time. However, it's wise not to make this a big issue, or your child will begin to see certain foods as forbidden—which will just enhance their appeal.

When you eat out in restaurants, you don't have to order food from a children's menu if all that offers is fried and processed choices (burger and french fries followed by ice cream, for instance). Order an adult starter or share a main dish with your child, or ask to substitute vegetables or a salad for the chips. Also ask for diluted juices instead of sodas.

Combating food fussiness is not as difficult as it might seem:

- Introduce a variety of foods as early as possible and set a good example.
- Remember, it's as much about psychology as nutrition. Be firm and consistent.

Chapter 23

Guerilla Tactics in the Supermarket

You'll have to face it sooner or later: what you want for your child and what the food manufacturers and marketers want are two different things. So you need to develop some guerrilla tactics in the supermarket, reading the labels carefully and reading between the lines. The hopeful news is that, these days, there really is plenty of choice even in mainstream supermarkets. Add in what health food stores have to offer, and it just isn't that difficult to fill pantry and refrigerator with wonderfully nutritious and delicious foods.

Here are the twelve golden shopping rules:

1. *Avoid foods that contain hydrogenated fats.*
   Check the label for the words "hydrogenated" and "vegetable oil." If it contains vegetable oil and has a long shelf life, the oil in the product has been hydrogenated—that is, processed so it hardens. As we discussed in chapter 3, hydrogenated fats interfere with the brain's use of essential fats and, ultimately, with the smooth working of the brain.

2. *Avoid foods that contain sugar.*
   Check labels for sugar, which includes sucrose, glucose, dextrose, maltose, and any other "-ose," as well as syrups such as corn and maple. Sugars that won't wreak havoc on your child's blood glucose include xylitol, fructose, and agave nectar, which is used in

drinks. Watch out for high-fructose corn syrup—it belongs to the syrup category despite its name! Only go for products where even these sugars are a long way down the ingredients list.

3. *Avoid processed juice and fruit juice drinks.*
   As discussed in chapter 1, processed fruit juices and fruit juice drinks are no better than sugary water. With these products, don't be fooled by the manufacturers' assertions that the drink has been fortified with vitamins and minerals. All this means is that the original and natural nutrients have been destroyed through processing. The only acceptable juices are freshly made ones, or the kind that's kept in the refrigerated case and has a very short shelf life—just a few days, maximum. Apple juice is the best choice since apples contain mainly fructose.

4. *Buy small blocks of cheese and small cartons of milk.*
   Consuming a lot of dairy products can potentially trigger a sensitivity to these foods—milk is one of the top allergens, after all. Most cheese also has a lot of saturated fat. If you and your children are eating dairy products, don't buy family-sized blocks of cheese and gallon containers of milk—unless you are a family of twenty! Buying smaller packages will keep your consumption down to a moderate level. Buy stronger-flavored cheeses such as Parmesan or mature Cheddar so that they can be used as a garnish rather than be eaten by the slab.

5. *Choose free-range, organic, and omega-3 rich eggs.*
   Eggs are a superb brain food, but they're only as healthy as the chicken who laid them. If you can, buy omega-3-enriched eggs, preferably organic or at least free-range.

6. *Avoid foods that contain additives, preservatives, and other chemicals.*
   Check the list of nasties in chapter 8, on page 75, and avoid these rigorously. As a good rule of thumb, a shorter ingredients list is likely to indicate a more wholesome food. For example, bread

may have as few as three ingredients or as many as thirty. Most important, if you read a long ingredients list and don't recognize many of these substances as food—that is, something that grew on a tree or in the ground, for example—or you feel you could better recognize and pronounce them if you had a chemistry degree, this should sound the alarm bell that this product is not a good thing to give your child.

7. *Make a list and stick to it.*
   A list is especially important if your child is going to the supermarket with you. You could write the list together. Use generic terms such as "fruits and veggies" so you're not limiting yourself and can pick what looks good. Don't put anything in the shopping cart that's not on the list, unless of course it's something you genuinely forgot you needed (and that clearly doesn't include chocolate cookies!). If you are strict about this, your child will accept it. Never give in to your child's demands and don't be afraid of a tantrum. Giving in teaches her that a tantrum gets her exactly what she wants. Avoid the cookie and candy aisles altogether. Remember, if she watches children's TV, every ad break is showcasing some refined, sugar-laden food that comes with small plastic gifts. Stay away from them!

8. *Eat before you go shopping.*
   And if your child is coming with you, give her a snack too. An apple and a few Brazil nuts in the car on the way to the supermarket will keep her blood sugar levels even. A snack deflects her cravings for sugary foods and also prevents the irritability that goes along with it. Take a bottle of water into the supermarket, too.

9. *Buy organic when you can.*
   Sometimes there is very little price difference between organic and nonorganic foods, which is great news. But be careful about organic processed foods. The ingredients are probably better quality, and they're likely to be free from additives, but organic

pizza and fries are still pizza and fries, and organic cake can still be laden with sugar. And as we've seen, refined carbohydrates add nothing to a healthful diet.

10. *Choose whole foods over refined and processed.*
Whole food means brown rice, whole-grain pasta, and whole grain bread instead of white. Choose whole vegetables, not ready-prepared vegetables—these will have been hemorrhaging nutrients since they were sliced. It's better, and much cheaper, to buy a whole lettuce or cabbage than to buy prepared salads or salad greens that start to wilt within minutes of opening the bag.

11. *Variety is the spice of life.*
Be adventurous and try new things, especially fresh produce. Have you ever eaten quinoa or pearl barley or had raw grated beets in a salad? Variety is key to good nutrition and makes mealtimes a lot more pleasurable, too.

12. *Watch out for "95 percent fat free."*
As we discussed in chapter 3, fat phobia is misguided. It's the *type* of fat that counts. Most products that claim to be low-fat have had sugar added to make them palatable, so they're not any better (and probably worse) than the original. Watch out for reduced-fat items where the original item is actually a naturally high-fat food. An example is low-fat butter. Butter is supposed to be virtually 100 percent fat, so check the ingredients list to see what's been added instead.

Chapter 24

Top Tips in the Kitchen

If your child has developed a taste for less-than-nutritious foods, you'll need to change his diet. Does even the idea fill you with foreboding? Don't worry: although it can be tough weaning him off double cheeseburgers and supersize fries, this chapter shows it can be done gradually and relatively painlessly, all around.

For example, if your child refuses to eat vegetables but will eat tomato sauce, begin by adding small amounts of pureed vegetables to the sauce and increase teaspoon by teaspoon over the days and weeks. This way, he simply won't notice the changing taste and appearance but within three months will actually be eating a highly nutritious, vitamin-rich sauce with his pasta. His taste buds will have become used to the vegetables. After this, it's simply a case of blending the vegetables less and less thoroughly so they get chunkier over time. When you finally present a plate of vegetables to your child, his taste buds will register them as a familiar food and he will be more likely to actually enjoy eating them.

For children who will eat only fish sticks and chicken nuggets, begin by making your own. Try to make them look similar to the commercial varieties. With these, too, you can begin to add pureed steamed vegetables, pureed boiled lentils, or pureed canned beans to the fish or chicken mixture. Add tiny amounts at the start, then increase gradually. Eventually, your child will be eating lentil and vegetable "sticks" and "nuggets" that are rich in nutrients and fiber instead of packaged food that may be of dubious quality and devoid of nutrients.

This is not to say that retraining taste buds isn't difficult. One of the biggest problems with getting kids who eat a lot of junk food to switch to healthful whole foods is the powerful artificial flavors and additives lurking in so many highly processed products. Whole foods can seem very bland by comparison at the start, but perseverance, the gradual introduction of wholesome ingredients as outlined above, and a clever use of herbs, spices, nutritious oils, lemon juice, and the like can work wonders.

Here are a few useful guidelines:

- If your child insists that he really doesn't like peas, for example, tell him he has to eat only three peas. (Although if he says this about every vegetable you serve, it's time to move on to the gradual-introduction method outlined above.)
- Steaming vegetables is the best cooking method. Steamed vegetables taste better and retain more nutrients than boiled, and are more nutritious than fried. Adding a drizzle of olive oil, a pat of butter, or a squeeze of lemon juice really boosts their flavor, too. Or you can steam-fry them—sauté the chosen vegetable briefly, add a tablespoon of soy sauce, water, or stock, then cover and cook until they're tender.
- Get your child involved in food preparation as early in life as possible. From a very young age, he can sprinkle seeds on a salad, for example.
- Many children will happily eat raw vegetables over cooked, so capitalize on this by providing raw veggies as predinner snacks.

So what, specifically, should you be feeding your child for optimum brain health?

THE BEST BREAKFASTS

To get your child off to the best start in the day, you can prepare wholesome versions of three basic options—cereal, cooked breakfast, or toast.

Cereal

The best cereal is oatmeal (cooked rolled oats or steel-cut oats, which are almost as good) or muesli (raw rolled oats) with plenty of nuts and seeds and fresh fruit (grated apple or diced ripe pear or plums are excellent).

Serve with dairy, soy, rice, oat, or nut milk. Watch out for boxed mueslis that are loaded with hidden sugar or a lot of dried fruit. Muesli shouldn't taste sweet. The sweetness comes from the fresh fruit you add.

Cooked Breakfast

Poached or scrambled eggs, perhaps with some smoked salmon, are excellent served with whole-grain bread. Choose whole loaves that most closely resemble a brick and have visible whole grains. Heavy and hard breads contain less yeast, which is better for blood sugar balance and also for digestive health. Some "brown" breads are brown only because of added coloring!

Toast

Again, heavy, grainy breads are the best choice. Rather than loads of sugary jellies or syrups, top with protein. You don't want to send your child out the door on a sugar high, only for him to slump an hour later in school. So give him hummus, avocado, or nut butters (almond, hazelnut, and cashew make a nice change from peanut, but whatever kind you go for, ensure it doesn't contain sweetener). Pumpkinseed butter is another supernutritious spread. The only jam your child should have should be sugar free and loaded with fruit, such as blueberries.

Unless your child is allergic to dairy, butter is a better choice than margarine or any of the other alternative spreads. If your child is allergic to dairy, then pumpkinseed butter or tahini (made from sesame seeds and their oil) are the best nondairy spreads.

LUNCH AND DINNER—THE TEMPLATE

With breakfast taken care of, how should you approach lunch and dinner? If you think of a plate and how to fill it, both of these meals should be about a quarter protein, a quarter starchy carbohydrates, and the remaining half vegetables and/or salad. Protein-rich foods are fish, eggs, meat, legumes (lentils and beans), quinoa, and nuts and seeds; starchy carbohydrates include bread, pasta, rice, potatoes, yams, and corn; and vegetables are all other non-starch produce, whether eaten cooked or raw. These proportions should apply whether the foods sit separately on the plate or are combined into a soup, stew, or main-course tossed salad.

If the protein doesn't include some essential fats from nuts, seeds, or oily fish, simply add some by drizzling a good-quality cold-pressed seed oil on the vegetables or salad, or sprinkling on a garnish of ground seeds. (See the next chapter for ideas on school lunches and how to fill your child's lunch box with zingy, supernutritious foods.)

Two-Day Menu

DAY ONE

Breakfast
Oatmeal with chopped plum and seeds

Snack
An apple and a handful of raw cashews

Lunch
Spaghetti with meat sauce containing pureed vegetables hidden in the sauce

Snack
Sugar snap peas and cherry tomatoes

Dinner
Fish, mashed potatoes, broccoli, and green beans

Drinks throughout the day
Diluted fresh fruit juice or water

DAY TWO

Breakfast
Whole-grain toast with almond butter

Snack
A pear and some pumpkinseeds

Lunch
Pasta shapes with a chicken and tomato sauce
Carrot and celery sticks

Snack
Oat cookie and a plum

Dinner
Stew with chickpeas and a variety of vegetables

Drinks throughout the day
Diluted fresh fruit juice or water

LAUDABLE LEGUMES

Legumes (lentils and beans) may not be a food you grew up with, but they certainly deserve a prominent place in your family's diet. A great source of protein, they also add fiber and important nutrients, help hormonal balance, and are economical to boot—helping offset some of the costs you may incur through buying organic, for instance. As cultures from India to Mexico know, lentils and beans are also delicious and wonderfully versatile to cook with. You can use them to enliven a wide range of soups, stews, salads, veggie burgers, veggie dips, and sandwich fillings—the list is endless.

Dried lentils are cooked in a mere 15 to 30 minutes, depending on variety. Beans and chickpeas can be bought in cans from any supermarket (look for those packed in water, without sugar or salt) and just need rinsing before use. Or, if you're really enthusiastic, you can buy them dried, soak them overnight, and simmer them for the time indicated on the package. Note that legumes need to be chewed thoroughly, as otherwise they can cause gas.

All legumes (excluding the split kind) can also be sprouted, making a tasty and amazingly nutritious addition to salads and sandwiches. As the sprouting process only takes three or four days, your child might enjoy growing some of your own food and experiencing the excitement of watching its progress day by day.

CHOOSING FATS AND OILS FOR COOKING

If you must fry, far and away the best cooking oil is coconut. Despite its white, fatty appearance at refrigerated or room temperature, coconut oil is a very healthful choice because it cannot be harmed by heating. The medium-chain triglycerides or MCTs it contains are also much easier for the body to burn for energy, so it's less likely to be stored as fat. And don't worry—it has no real flavor of its own. The next best option is butter, unless you're dairy free, followed by olive oil (a monounsaturated fat), which is slightly damaged by frying.

Whichever fat you use, never fry at high heat. Steam-frying is much better, as we've seen. Sauté onions and garlic in your chosen oil just enough to generate heat and soften slightly, then add the other ingredients and a dash of water, stock, or soy sauce. Cover and steam gently for a few minutes. With this method, the temperature and the nutrient loss are much lower.

And if you want to give soups, stews, and curries a rich, creamy touch, you don't have to go for cream; coconut milk or a dab of hummus or tahini is a wholesome dairy-free option.

Chapter 25

Making Healthful Meals in School Cool

Once your child starts attending school, or spends time with a babysitter, your control of her diet begins to slip away. Essentially, your child will either be eating the packed lunch that you supply or a school meal. Things are improving there, spurred on by campaigns such as that of Alice Waters and her Chez Panisse Foundation, along with government recognition that stemming the obesity epidemic must start with the youngest Americans. But there's no way around it: you still need to be sure of what your child is eating when you're not around.

AT NURSERY SCHOOL OR SCHOOL

It's particularly important to check out preschools, because young children aren't really up to making a lot of choices about food. Before you commit to one, find out what they will be feeding your child. If it doesn't impress you as nutritious, look elsewhere or see if they're in the process of doing something about it. If parents demand better food for their children, it will be provided—there's nothing as effective for change as voting with your choices.

In school, however, what a child eats is likely to be completely up to her. If your child already has an appetite for wholesome food, then she is more likely to make good choices. If not, then it is doubly important that the choices offered are good.

We find that when working with children who choose their own lunch in school, it's important that they have a good incentive to eat wholesome food. Prevention of heart disease in later life is unlikely to impress a ten-year-old much; that's just too far into the future for her to be able to care about. But if you tell her it will help her be a better tennis player, have more friends, do better in class, stop getting into trouble, and have clear skin, that's much more motivating.

Optimum nutrition improves health and well-being on myriad levels, but you need to focus on what's important to your child. After all, being better at math is not much of an incentive to an artistic child who has no interest in math.

Breakfast in School

Eating breakfast in school is great in theory, but you'll need to take a good look at what's on the menu before you allow your child to go for it. If breakfast is sugary cereal, doughnuts, white toast, maple syrup, and juice drinks, you're effectively putting your child on a blood sugar roller coaster. So you have two choices: exert your influence as a concerned parent to ensure that better breakfast options (outlined in chapter 24) are available, or give your child breakfast at home.

The Optimum Lunch Box and Snacks

When you're putting your child's lunch box and snacks together for the day, follow the lunch and dinner templates on page 200, as these supply the best range of nutrients and best blood sugar balance. A couple of peanut butter sandwiches on whole-grain bread with a simple salad fits the bill.

A salad box is a great alternative to sandwiches in summer, but make sure it contains enough protein and quality carbohydrates. An active child cannot get through the day on lettuce leaves. Try tuna and pasta salad with carrot and celery sticks and some sugar snap peas; or falafel or lentil burgers with brown basmati rice salad and cherry tomatoes, baby corn, and sprouts. In winter, a thermos of thick, hearty soup is wonderful—just be sure to follow the proportions in the lunch and dinner template when you're making it.

Great snacks include fresh fruit, nuts and seeds, oatcake crackers, raw vegetables, or savory muffins (made with chickpea flour, for example). As for drinks, it seems most children will drink water quite happily if it's in a sport bottle, so pop in one of those full of water or diluted fruit juice each day.

So, to recap—what might go into that packed lunch? Try a hummus and salad sandwich on whole-grain rye bread or a peanut butter sandwich on whole-grain bread, some carrot sticks, an apple, some Brazil nuts, a couple of oatcake crackers, and a bottle of water.

ON THE WAY TO AND FROM SCHOOL

Once your child has her own money and is walking to school on her own, you can't stop her from buying candy at the store on the way to or from school. However, if her schoolbag is full of delicious, wholesome snacks and her pockets are not full of money, you will have less to worry about. Also, if she's had a good breakfast at home, she'll be less inclined to buy food on the way to school. And if she's used to nutritious, wholesome food and has balanced blood sugar, she will be less inclined to gorge on the really unwholesome stuff.

So keep a check on it, but try not to make it a big deal. On the whole, the food your child eats will be what you provide for her at home, and that is what's most important.

Chapter 26

Supplements for Superkids

We've demonstrated throughout this book that a varied and nutritious diet is the keystone of good mental and emotional health. But sometimes even the best diets fail to provide appropriate levels of all the nutrients we need, and some children need more of certain nutrients than others. Also, as we've seen, children can be very picky eaters. Add to that the logistical challenge of providing a day's meals perfectly balanced in every nutrient, and what you're looking at is supplements.

Supplementation is the most reliable way to ensure your child gets appropriate levels of all the vitamins and minerals he needs to be optimally nourished; this is even more important if your child is having a hard time of it mentally or emotionally. Remember that there's a range of vitamins and minerals essential for good health, and a small deficiency in any one nutrient could have a serious impact on your growing child.

WHEN TO START SUPPLEMENTING

As soon as you start weaning your child, it's worth supplementing. As long as you're breast-feeding, it's you who needs to take the supplemental nutrients, which then get passed on to your child naturally.

The following chart (parts of which also appear in chapter 11) shows the ideal daily amounts of vitamins, minerals, and essential fats to supplement from weaning to age thirteen, assuming you are feeding your child a reasonably nutritious diet. Once a child is fourteen, adult supplementation applies. You can determine the right amounts using chapter 45 of the *New Optimum Nutrition Bible,* or see www.patrickholford.com/content .asp?id_Content=1206.

The Ideal Daily Supplement Program

Age	Unit	Less than 1	1-2	3-4	5-6	7-8	9-11	12-13
Nutrient								
Essential Vitamins								
A (retinol) *	mcg	500	650	800	1,000	1,500	2,000	2,500
D*	mcg	3	4	5	7	9	11	12
E*	mg	13	16	20	23	30	40	50
C	mg	100	150	300	400	500	600	700
B1 (thiamine)	mg	5	6	8	12	16	20	24
B2 (riboflavin)	mg	5	6	8	12	16	20	24
B3 (niacin)	mg	7	12	16	18	20	22	24
B5 (pantothenic acid)	mg	10	15	20	25	30	35	40
B6 (pyridoxine)	mg	5	7	10	12	16	20	25
B12	mcg	5	6.5	8	9	10	10	10
Folic acid	mcg	100	120	140	160	180	200	220
Biotin	mcg	30	45	60	70	80	90	100
Essential Minerals								
Calcium	mg	150	165	180	190	200	210	220
Magnesium	mg	50	65	80	90	100	110	120
Iron	mg	4	5.5	7	8	9	10	10
Zinc	mg	4	5.5	7	8	9	10	10
Manganese	mcg	300	350	400	500	700	1,000	1,000
Iodine	mcg	40	50	60	70	80	90	100
Chromium	mcg	15	19	23	25	27	30	30
Selenium	mcg	10	18	20	24	26	28	30
Copper	mcg	400	550	700	800	900	1,000	1,000

* To calculate IU values, please see conversions on page viii.   *(continued)*

The Ideal Daily Supplement Program, continued

Age	Less than 1	1	2	3–4	5–6	7–8	9–11
Essential Fats							
GLA	50 mg	75	95	110	135	135	135
EPA	100 mg	175	250	300	350	350	350
DHA	100 mg	140	175	200	225	225	225
Other Brain Nutrients (optional)							
Phosphatidylcholine	250 to 400 mg						
Phosphatidylserine	20 to 45 mg						
DMAE	200 to 300 mg						
Glutamine	250 to 1,000 mg						
Pyroglutamate	300 to 450 mg						
Trimethylglycine (TMG)	250 to 1,000 mg						

CHOOSING THE RIGHT SUPPLEMENTS

With supplements for your child, you're looking at three broad areas: multivitamins, essential fats, and, if needed, extra brain nutrients.

Finding a Good Multivitamin

Many companies formulate single multivitamin and mineral supplements that incorporate all the necessary nutrients especially for children (see Resources, page 219). The chart above will give you guidelines on the levels of nutrients to look for. You can choose chewable (or crushable in the early stages) or liquid or soluble formulas, depending on your (or your child's) preferences.

A common problem that parents find with supplements is that they may be lacking in adequate calcium, magnesium, and zinc. There are a number of ways to get around this problem. Assuming you are giving your child ground seeds every day, as we recommend, these will guarantee a reasonable amount of calcium, magnesium, and zinc. You can get powdered calcium and magnesium to add to drinks, or a chewable vitamin C that uses calcium and magnesium ascorbate, thus killing three birds with one stone. If your child doesn't sleep well and a little extra magnesium would help, this is a good option. The best way to give your child a little extra vitamin C is to make sure he eats at least five servings of fruit and vegetables a day. The best foods for vitamin C are bell peppers, broccoli, berries, and citrus fruit.

You should ideally give your child his supplement with breakfast, and certainly not last thing at night, as the B vitamins can have a mild stimulatory effect. (For some children, glutamine can also be stimulating.) Children also tend to be more susceptible to vitamin toxicity than adults, and while the doses listed are well within any potentially toxic limits for even the most sensitive child, don't be tempted to give much more than these recommended levels unless under the direction and supervision of a nutritionist.

Essential Fats to Boost IQ

As long as your child is eating oily fish three times a week and a daily portion of seeds, he should be getting a good background level of essential fats to help his brain develop and boost IQ. However, if he doesn't eat fish or doesn't have seeds every day, we recommend you supplement his diet with an essential fat formula. Look for one that contains both GLA (omega-6) and DHA and EPA, which are the most important omega-3 fats for development. The most important essential fat is omega-3, and there are many different forms of supplements supplying this essential fat on the market, ranging from pastes to drinks to small capsules. You can always pierce a capsule and add it to juice or food.

The preceding chart gives you the rough quantities to aim for in a supplement, assuming your child is receiving the same again from seeds and the occasional serving of oily fish.

Extra Brain Nutrients

In addition to the essential vitamins, minerals, and fats, we've also extolled the virtues of phospholipids (phosphatidylcholine, phosphatidylserine, and DMAE), as well as glutamine and its cousin pyroglutamate. These can be supplemented as well, but they usually come in tablets that might be hard for a younger child to swallow. For phosphatidylcholine (PC), you can add some lecithin granules to cereal, generally giving 2 teaspoons of regular lecithin or 1 teaspoon of high-phosphatidylcholine lecithin. Glutamine also comes in a powder that easily dissolves in water or diluted juice.

To ensure your child is getting enough brain-boosting nutrients, there are several easy steps you can take:

- Give your child a good multivitamin and mineral formula based on the nutrient levels in this chapter.
- Give your child an omega-3 fish oil supplement every day.
- If your child is struggling, look for a specific brain food formula with the additional brain nutrients listed above.

Chapter 27

Join the Food for the Brain Campaign

I t's in childhood that we build the rest of our lives—yet it sometimes seems as if there are too many pitfalls on this journey. You have no doubt despaired at the quality of school meals, the junk designed to fill kids' lunch boxes, and the vast, ever-expanding variety of sugary drinks and snacks crowding the supermarket shelves. You've probably wondered why something as important as optimum nutrition isn't taught in schools so all children can learn how what they eat affects their health and their minds. You've no doubt wondered why legislators aren't doing more to act on the obvious link between poor diet and increasing behavioral problems and crime.

Every year, enormous sums are spent at both federal and state level on additional support for children with learning and behavioral problems, but so far nutrition is entirely overlooked. You might wish there were a way you could make a difference, and there is:

1. Nutritious eating starts at home. Get your own diet and your child's on track by following the advice in this book.

2. Have a close look at the food your child is served in school and find out how much choice she has. For example, is she free to choose to eat a lunch of french fries every day?

3. Speak to the person responsible for nutrition in your child's
    school. Find out why the school chooses to serve the food that
    they do. Give them a copy of this book. Join the PTA and put
    optimum nutrition for children's minds on the agenda.

4. Find local nonprofit organizations working toward the
    same goals. For example, have a look at the website of the
    Healthy School Food Coalition in Los Angeles, California
    (http://departments.oxy.edu/uepi/cfj/hsfcoalition.htm) or
    the NY Coalition for Healthy School Food (www.healthylunches
    .org/index.htm).

5. Encourage the parents in your child's school to complete
    the free online Food for the Brain Child Questionnaire,
    which will give you a report identifying simple nutritional
    changes that are likely to help your child the most. Visit
    www.foodforthebrain.org, a UK-based website that has lots
    of useful information for parents and schools.

Above all, remember: You are not alone. More and more parents like
you, teachers, schools, doctors, politicians, and children are waking up to
the fact that what you eat has a profound effect not only on your physical health, but also on how you think and feel. By joining the campaign,
you're helping create a better world in the future for our children, and our
children's children.

Wishing you health and happiness,

—Patrick Holford and Deborah Colson

Recommended Reading

Braly, James, and Patrick Holford. *Hidden Food Allergies: The Essential Guide to Uncovering Hidden Food Allergies—and Achieving Permanent Relief.* Basic Health Publications, 2006.

Colborn, Theo, Dianne Dumanoski, and John Peter Meyers. *Our Stolen Future.* Penguin Books, 1997.

Cooper, Ann, and Lisa M. Holmes. *Lunch Lessons: Changing the Way We Feed Our Children.* HarperCollins, 2006.

Crawford, M., and O. Marsh. *Nutrition and Evolution.* Keats, 1995.

Erasmus, Udo. *Fats that Heal, Fats that Kill.* Alive Books, 1994.

Evers, Connie Liakos. *How to Teach Nutrition to Kids.* 24 Carrot Press, 2003.

Holford, Patrick. *Optimum Nutrition for the Mind.* Basic Health Publications, 2004.

Holford, Patrick. *The New Optimum Nutrition Bible.* Crossing Press, 2005.

Holford, Patrick, and Fiona McDonald Joyce. *Smart Foods for Smart Kids.* Piatkus Books, 2007.

Holford, Patrick, and Susannah Lawson. *Optimum Nutrition Before, During and After Pregnancy.* Piatkus Books, 2004.

Lapine, Missy Chase. *The Sneaky Chef: Simple Strategies for Hiding Healthy Foods in Kids' Favorite Meals.* Running Press, 2007.

Resources

SERVICES AND ASSOCIATIONS

Autism Research Institute (ARI)

The Autism Research Institute, founded by Bernard Rimland, PhD, is the hub of a worldwide network of parents and professionals concerned with autism. The only organization of its kind, ARI was founded in 1967 to conduct and foster scientific research designed to improve the methods of diagnosing, treating, and preventing autism. ARI also disseminates research findings to parents and others all over the world who are seeking help. The ARI data bank, the world's largest, contains nearly 25,000 detailed case histories of autistic children from over sixty countries.

AUTISM RESEARCH INSTITUTE
4182 Adams Avenue
San Diego, CA 92116
(866) 366-3361
www.autism.com/ari

Brain Bio Centre

The Brain Bio Centre is an outpatient clinical treatment center specializing in the optimum nutrition approach to mental health problems. The center offers comprehensive assessment of biochemical imbalances that can contribute to mental health problems and advice on how to correct these imbalances as a means to restore health.

www.brainbiocentre.com

Food for the Brain

Food for the Brain is a nonprofit foundation set up to promote the link between optimum nutrition and mental health. The Food for the Brain Schools Campaign also gives advice to schools and parents on how to make kids smarter by improving the quality of food inside and outside of school. It has free e-news, a library of research, and special reports on subjects such as autism. It also has a free online Food for the Brain Child Questionnaire that gives you a report on what simple changes will help your child the most.

www.foodforthebrain.org

International Dyslexia Association (IDA)

The International Dyslexia Association is a 501(c)(3) nonprofit scientific and educational organization dedicated to the study and treatment of the learning disability dyslexia, as well as related language-based learning differences. The association has forty-seven branches throughout the United States and Canada.

INTERNATIONAL DYSLEXIA ASSOCIATION
40 York Road
4th Floor
Baltimore, MD 21204
(410) 296-0232
www.interdys.org

International Society of Orthomolecular Medicine

The International Society of Orthomolecular Medicine exists to further the advancement of orthomolecular medicine throughout the world, and to unite the many and various groups already operating in eighteen countries. Orthomolecular medicine is the practice of using the most appropriate nutrients, including vitamins, minerals, and other essential compounds, in the most therapeutic amounts, according to an individual's particular biochemical requirements to establish optimum health.

www.orthomed.org

National Gardening Association

The National Gardening Association runs a website called Kids Gardening. Here they have plenty of helpful information and teaching resources for parents and teachers on getting your kids involved in gardening both at home and in school. Research clearly shows that kids will eat vegetables much more willingly if they grow them themselves!

NATIONAL GARDENING ASSOCIATION
1100 Dorset Street
South Burlington, VT 05403
(800) 538-7476 (800-LETSGRO)
www.kidsgardening.com

PatrickHolford.com

One of the most visited nutrition website in the world, www.patrickholford
.com contains many useful articles and information on optimum nutrition
for your child. Patrick Holford also writes a bimonthly newsletter and free
e-news to help keep you informed. There's a free online 100% Health Check
that measures your health and identifies the key areas to address to effect
your own health transformation.

www.patrickholford.com

Pfeiffer Treatment Center

The Pfeiffer Treatment Center (PTC) is a private, nonprofit clinic that provides extensive biochemical analysis and individualized nutrient-based
treatment to both children and adults. PTC specializes in treating learning and behavior problems, such as ADD and ADHD, and developmental
disorders, such as autism. PTC is staffed by a team of physicians, chemists,
and other professionals who specialize in the effects of biochemistry on
behavior, thought, and mood.

PFEIFFER TREATMENT CENTER
4575 Weaver Parkway
Warrenville, IL 60555
(630) 505-0300
www.hriptc.org

Safe Harbor

Safe Harbor is a nonprofit corporation that sponsors a website for those
interested in alternative and nutritional approaches to mental health. The
website offers a free e-news letter and other useful services, including
information on finding an alternative mental health practitioner.

www.alternativementalhealth.com

Nutrition Consultations

One-on-one nutrition consultations are available through naturopathic physicians, nutritionists, and physicians trained in the optimum nutrition approach. The following organizations can help you find a practitioner in your area.

AMERICAN ASSOCIATION FOR HEALTH FREEDOM
4620 Lee Highway
Suite 210
Arlington, VA 22207
(800) 230-2762
www.apma.net

AMERICAN ASSOCIATION OF NATUROPATHIC PHYSICIANS
4435 Wisconsin Avenue NW
Suite 403
Washington, DC 20016
(866) 538-2267
www.naturopathic.org

AMERICAN COLLEGE FOR ADVANCEMENT IN MEDICINE
24411 Ridge Route
Suite 115
Laguna Hills, CA 92653
(888) 439-6891
www.acam.org

AMERICAN HOLISTIC MEDICAL ASSOCIATION
1 Eagle Valley Court
Suite 201
Broadview Heights, OH 44147
(440) 838-1010
www.holisticmedicine.org

METAGENICS
100 Ave La Pata
San Clemente, CA 92673
(800) 962-9400
www.metagenics.com

TESTS

Laboratory tests are available for all the tests mentioned in this book, through nutritionists. Leading laboratories include the following.

Genova Diagnostics

Offers a urine test for IAG, hair analysis for heavy metal toxicity, and homocysteine test for vitamin B deficiencies.

> GENOVA DIAGNOSTICS
> 63 Zillicoa Street
> Asheville, NC 28801-1074
> (800) 522-4762
> www.genovadiagnostics.com

Immuno Laboratories

Offers IgE and IgG food allergy testing.

> IMMUNO LABORATORIES
> 6801 Powerline Road
> Fort Lauderdale, FL 33309
> (800) 231-9197
> www.immunolabs.com

Vitamin Diagnostics

Offers a urinary HPL test.

> VITAMIN DIAGNOSTICS
> Route 35, Industrial Drive
> Cliffwood Beach, NJ 07735
> (732) 583-7773

York Nutritional Laboratories

York Nutritional Laboratories offers a wide range of tests and specializes in testing that utilizes finger-prick blood samples that can be carried out at home. Includes the IgG ELISA (food intolerance) test.

> (888) 751-3388
> www.yorkallergyusa.com

SUPPLEMENTS

Enzymatic Therapy

The website has a "where to buy" function for retail stores and online e-stores.

(800) 783-2286

www.enzy.com

Nature's Plus

The website has a store locator.

www.naturesplus.com

Solgar Vitamin and Herb

The website has a "where to buy" function for retail stores and online e-stores.

(877) 765-4274 (877-SOLGAR-4)

www.solgar.com

Source Naturals

The website has a "where to buy" function for retail stores and online e-stores.

(800) 815-2333

www.sourcenaturals.com

Twinlab Corporation

The website gives product information only.

(800) 645-5626

www.twinlab.com

Endnotes

Introduction

1. D. Benton and G. Roberts, "Effect of Vitamin and Mineral Supplementation on Intelligence of School Children," *Lancet* 1, no. 8578 (1988): 140–43.

2. B. Lozoff et al., "Double Burden of Iron Deficiency in Infancy and Low Socioeconomic Status," *Archives of Pediatric & Adolescent Medicine* 160 (2006): 1108–13.

3. B. Gesch, "Influence of Supplementary Vitamins, Minerals and Essential Fats on the Antisocial Behavior of Young Adult Prisoners," *British Journal of Psychiatry* 181 (2002): 22–28

4. A. J. Richardson and P. Montgomery, "The Oxford-Durham Study: A Randomized Controlled Trial of Dietary Supplementation with Fatty Acids in Children with Developmental Coordination Disorder," *Pediatrics* 115 (2005): 1360–66.

5. A. K. Borjel et al., "Plasma Homocysteine Levels, MTHFR Polymorphisms, and School Achievement in a Population Sample of Swedish Children," *Haematologica Reports* 1, no. 3 (2005) 4.

6. C. M. Carter et al., "Effects of a Few Food Diet in Attention Deficit Disorder," *Archives of Disease in Childhood* 69 (1993): 564–68.

Chapter 1

1. World Health Organization, *The World Health Report 2001—Mental Health: New Understanding, New Hope* (WHO, 2001), available at www.who.int/whr/2001/.

2. A. K. Borjel et al., "Plasma Homocysteine Levels, MTHFR Polymorphisms 677C>T, 1298A>C, 1793G>A, and School Achievement in a Population Sample of Swedish Children" (paper presented at Homocysteine Metabolism, 5th International Conference, Milano, Italy, June 26–30, 2005).

3. J. Penland, "Zinc and Other Mineral Nutrients Related to Cognition and Behavior" (paper presented at Experimental Biology conference, San Diego, April 4, 2005, pending publication).

Chapter 2

1. A. G. Schauss, "Nutrition and Behavior," *Journal of Applied Nutrition* 35, no. 1 (1983): 30–35.

2. D. Benton et al., "The Impact of the Supply of Glucose to the Brain on Mood and Memory," *Nutrition Review* 59 no. 1, pt. 2 (2001): S20–S21.

3. AGGRESSION: D. Benton et al., "Mild Hypoglycaemia and Questionnaire Measures of Aggression," *Biological Psychology* 14, nos. 1–2 (1982): 129–35; A. Roy et al., "Monoamines, Glucose Metabolism, Aggression toward Self and Others," *International Journal of Neuroscience* 41, nos. 3–4 (1988): 261–64; A. G. Schauss, *Diet, Crime and Delinquency* (Parker House, 1980); M. Virkkunen, "Reactive Hypoglycaemic Tendency among Arsonists," *Acta Psychiatrica Scandinavica* 69, no. 5 (1984): 445–52; M. Virkkunen and S. Narvanen, "Tryptophan and Serotonin Levels during the Glucose Tolerance Test among Habitually Violent and Impulsive Offenders," *Neuropsychobiology* 17, nos. 1–2 (1987): 19–23; J. Yaryura-Tobias and F. Neziroglu, "Violent Behavior, Brain Dysrythmia and Glucose Dysfunction: A New Syndrome," *American Journal of Orthopsychiatry* 4 (1975): 182–85. ANXIETY: M. Bruce and M. Lader, "Caffeine Abstention and the Management of Anxiety Disorders," *Psychological Medicine* 19 (1989): 211–14; W. Wendel and W. Beebe, "Glycolytic Activity in Schizophrenia," in *Orthomolecular Psychiatry*, ed. D. Hawkins and L. Pauling (W. H. Freeman, 1973). HYPERACTIVITY AND ATTENTION DEFICIT: R. Prinz and D. Riddle, "Associations between Nutrition and Behavior in 5-Year-Old Children," *Nutrition Review* 43, suppl. (1986): 151-58. DEPRESSION: L. Christensen, "Psychological Distress and Diet—Effects of Sucrose and Caffeine," *Journal of Applied Nutrition* 40 (1988): 44–50. EATING DISORDERS: D. Fullerton et al., "Sugar, Opionoids and Binge Eating," *Brain Research Bulletin* 14, no. 6 (1985): 273–80. FATIGUE: L. Christensen, "Psychological Distress and Diet: Effects of Sucrose and Caffeine," *Journal of Applied Nutrition* 40 (1988): 44–50. LEARNING DIFFICULTIES: M. Colgan and L. Colgan, "Do Nutrient Supplements and Dietary Changes Affect Learning and Emotional Reactions of Children with Learning Difficulties? A Controlled Series of 16 Cases," *Nutrition and Health* 3 (1984): 69–77; J. Goldman et al., "Behavioral Effects of Sucrose on Preschool Children," *Journal of Abnormal Child Psychology* 14, no. 4 (1986): 565–77; M. Lester et al., "Refined Carbohydrate Intake, Hair Cadmium Levels and Cognitive Functioning in Children," *Nutrition and Behavior* 1 (1982): 3–13; S. Schoenthaler et al., "The Impact of Low Food Additive and Sucrose Diet on Academic Performance

in 803 New York City Public Schools," *International Journal of Biosocial and Medical Research* 8, no. 2 (1986): 185–95.

4. R. J. Prinz et al., "Dietary Correlates of Hyperactive Behavior in Children," *Journal of Consulting and Clinical Psychology* 48 (1980): 760–69; S. J. Schoenthaler et al., "The Effect of Randomised Vitamin-Mineral Supplementation on Violent and Non-violent Antisocial Behaviour among Incarcerated Juveniles," *Journal of Nutritional & Environmental Medicine* 7 (1997): 343–52.

5. L. Langseth and J. Dowd, "Glucose Tolerance and Hyperkinesis," *Food and Cosmetics Toxicology* 16 (1978): 129.

6. R. G. Walton et al., "Adverse Reactions to Aspartame: Double Blind Challenge in Patients from a Vulnerable Population," *Journal of Biological Psychiatry* 34, nos. 1–2 (1993): 13–17.

7. K. A. Wesnes et al., "Breakfast Reduces Declines in Attention and Memory over the Morning in Schoolchildren," *Appetite* 41 (2003): 329–31.

8. K. Gilliland and D. Andress, "Ad Lib Caffeine Consumption, Symptoms of Caffeinism, and Academic Performance," *American Journal of Psychiatry* 138, no. 4 (1981): 512–14.

9. N. J. Richardson et al., "Mood and Performance Effects of Caffeine in Relation to Acute and Chronic Caffeine Deprivation," *Pharmacology, Biochemistry and Behavior* 52, no. 2 (1995): 313–20.

Chapter 3

1. M. Makrides et al., "Are Long-Chain Polyunsaturated Fatty Acids Essential Nutrients in Infancy?' *Lancet* 345 (1995): 1463–68; L. Stevens, "Essential Fat Metabolism in Boys with Attention-Deficit Hyperactivity Disorder," *American Journal of Clinical Nutrition* 62 (1995): 761–68.

2. P. Willatts et al., "Effect of Long-Chain Polyunsaturated Fatty Acids in Infant Formula on Problem Solving at 10 Months of Age," *Lancet* 352 (1998): 688–91.

3. J. B. Helland et al., "Maternal Supplementation with Very-Long-Chain N-3 Fatty Acids during Pregnancy and Lactation Augments Children's IQ at 4 Years of Age," *Pediatrics* 111 (2003): 39–44.

4. A. Richardson and B. Puri, "A Randomized Double-Blind, Placebo-Controlled Study of the Effects of Supplementation with Highly Unsaturated Fatty Acids on ADHD-Related Symptoms in Children with Specific Learning Difficulties," *Progress in Neuro-Psychopharmacology & Biological Psychiatry* 26, no. 2 (2002): 233–39.

5. A. J. Richardson and P. Montgomery, "The Oxford-Durham Study: A Randomized Controlled Trial of Dietary Supplementation with Fatty Acids in Children with Developmental Coordination Disorder," *Pediatrics* 115 (2005): 1360–66.

6. L. J. Stevens et al., "Essential Fat Metabolism in Boys with Attention-Deficit Hyperactivity Disorder," *American Journal of Clinical Nutrition* 65 (1995): 761–68.

7. J. R. Burgess, "ADHD: Observational and Interventional Studies" (NIH Workshop on Omega-3 EFAs in Psychiatric Disorders, National Institutes of Health, Bethesda, MD, 1988); A. J. Richardson et al., "Treatment with Highly Unsaturated Fatty Acids Can Reduce ADHD Symptoms in Children with Specific Learning Difficulties: A Randomised Controlled Trial" (paper given at British Dyslexia Association International Conference, University of York, UK, April 2001); A. Richardson and B. Puri, "A Randomized Double-Blind, Placebo-Controlled Study of the Effects of Supplementation with Highly Unsaturated Fatty Acids on ADHD-Related Symptoms in Children with Specific Learning Difficulties," *Progress in Neuro-Psychopharmacology & Biological Psychiatry* 26, no. 2 (2002): 233–39.

8. S. E. Carlson et al., "Long-Term Feeding of Formulas High in Linolenic Acid and Marine Oil to Very Low Birth Weight Infants: Phospholipid Fatty Acids," *Pediatric Research* 30 (1991): 404–12.

9. A. J. Richardson and P. Montgomery, "The Oxford-Durham Study," *Pediatrics* 115, no. 5 (2005): 1360-66.

Chapter 4

1. G. Pyapali et al., "Prenatal Dietary Choline Supplementation," *Journal of Neurophysiology* 79, no. 4 (1998): 1790–96; W. H. Meck et al., "Perinatal Choline Supplementation Increases the Threshold for Chunking in Spatial Memory," *Neuroreport* 8 (1997): 3053–59.

2. S. Y. Chung et al., "Administration of Phosphatidylcholine Increases Brain Acetylcholine Concentration and Improves Memory in Mice with Dementia," *Journal of Nutrition* 125, no. 6 (1995): 1484–89.

3. R. J. Wurtman and S. H. Zeisel, "Brain Choline: Its Sources and Effects on the Synthesis and Release of Acetylcholine," *Aging* 19 (1982): 303–13.

Chapter 5

1.　W. Poldinger et al., "A Functional-Dimensional Approach to Depression: Serotonin Deficiency and Target Syndrome in a Comparison of 5-Hydroxytryptophan and Fluvoxamine," *Psychopathology* 24, no. 2 (1991): 53–81; J. B. Deijen et al., "Tyrosine Improves Cognitive Performance and Reduces Blood Pressure in Cadets," *Brain Research Bulletin* 48, no. 2 (1999): 203–9; I. S. Shiah and N. Yatham, "GABA Functions in Mood Disorders: An Update and Critical Review," *Nature Life Sciences* 63, no. 15 (1998): 1289–303.

2.　U.S. Food and Drug Administration, "FDA Proposes New Warnings about Suicidal Thinking, Behavior in Young Adults Who Take Antidepressant Medications," *FDA News* P07-77 (May 2, 2007), www.fda.gov/bbs/topics/NEWS/2007/NEW01624.html.

Chapter 6

1.　D. Benton and G. Roberts, "Effect of Vitamin and Mineral Supplementation on Intelligence of a Sample of School Children," *Lancet* 1, no. 8578 (1998): 140–43.

2.　A. Lucas et al., "Randomised Trial of Early Diet in Preterm Babies and Later Intelligence Quotient," *British Medical Journal* 317 (1998): 1481–87.

3.　A. K. Borjel et al., "Plasma Homocysteine Levels, MTHFR Polymorphisms, and School Achievement in a Population Sample of Swedish Children," *Haematologica Reports* 1, no. 3 (2005) 4.

4.　D. Benton et al., "The Impact of Long-Term Vitamin Supplementation on Cognitive Functioning," *Journal of Psychopharmacology* (Berl) 117, no. 3 (1995): 298–305; D. Benton et al., "Thiamine Supplementation, Mood and Cognitive Functioning," *Journal of Psychopharmacology* (Berl) 129, no. 1 (1997): 66–71.

5.　M. Louwman et al., "Signs of Impaired Cognitive Function in Adolescents with Marginal Cobalamin Status," *American Journal of Clinical Nutrition* 72 (2000): 762–69.

6.　J. Greenblatt et al., "Folic Acid in Neurodevelopment and Child Psychiatry Progress," *Neuro-Psychopharmacology & Biological Psychiatry* 18, no. 4 (1994): 647–60.

7.　R. R. Briefel et al., "Zinc Intake of the U.S. Population: Findings from the Third National Health and Nutrition Examination Survey 1988–1994," *Journal of Nutrition* 130 (2000): 1367S–73S.

8. S. Johnson, "Micronutrient Accumulation and Depletion in Schizophrenia, Epilepsy, Autism and Parkinson's Disease?" *Medical Hypotheses* 56, no. 5 (2002): 641–45.

9. J. Penland, "Zinc Affects Cognition and Psychosocial Function of Middle-School Children" (paper presented at Experimental Biology conference, San Diego, April 4, 2005, pending publication).

Chapter 7

1. H. L. Needleman et al., "The Long-Term Effects of Exposure to Low Doses of Lead in Childhood: An 11-Year Follow-Up Report," *New England Journal of Medicine* 332 (1990): 83–88.

Chapter 8

1. E. M. Haas with B. Levin, *Staying Healthy with Nutrition* (Celestial Arts, 2006).

2. N. I. Ward et al., "The Influence of the Chemical Additive Tartrazine on the Zinc Status of Hyperactive Children—A Double-Blind Placebo Controlled Study," *Journal of Nutritional Medicine* 1 (1990): 51–57.

3. B. Bateman et al., "The Effects of a Double Blind, Placebo Controlled, Artificial Food Colourings and Benzoate Preservative Challenge on Hyperactivity in a General Population Sample of Preschool Children," *Archives of Disease in Childhood* 89 (2004): 506–11.

4. D. McCann et al., "Food Additives and Hyperactive Behavior in 3-Year-Old and 8/9-Year-Old Children in the Community: A Randomised, Double-Blinded, Placebo-Controlled Trial," *Lancet* 370, no. 9598 (2007): 1560–67.

Chapter 9

1. E. Young et al., "A Population Study of Food Intolerance," *Lancet* 343 (1994): 1127–29; British Society for Allergy and Environmental Medicine, *Effective Allergy Practice* (1984).

2. T. Randolph, "Allergy as a Causative Factor of Fatigue, Irritability and Behavior Problems of Children," *Journal of Pediatrics* 31 (1947): 560; A. Rowe, "Allergic Toxemia and Fatigue," *Annals of Allergy, Asthma & Immunology* 17 (1959): 9; F. Speer, ed., "Etiology: Foods," in *Allergy of the Nervous System* (Charles C. Thomas, 1970); M. Campbell, "Neurologic Manifestations of Allergic Disease,"

Annals of Allergy, Asthma & Immunology 31 (1973): 485; K. Hall, "Allergy of the Nervous System: A Review," *Annals of Allergy, Asthma & Immunology* 36 (1976): 49–64; V. Pippere, "Some Varieties of Food Intolerance in Psychiatric Patients," *Nutrition and Health* 3, no. 3 (1984): 125–36; C. Pfeiffer and P. Holford, *Mental Illness and Schizophrenia: The Nutrition Connection* (Thorsons, 1989); T. Tuormaa, *An Alternative to Psychiatry* (The Book Guild, 1991).

3.   J. Egger et al., "Controlled Trial of Oligoantigenic Treatment in the Hyperkinetic Syndrome," *Lancet* 1, no. 8428 (1985): 540–45.

4.   J. Egger et al., "Is Migraine a Food Allergy? A Double-Blind Controlled Trial of Oligoantigenic Diet Treatment," *Lancet* 2, no. 8355 (1983): 865–69.

Chapter 11

1.   A. L. Kubala and M. M. Katz, "Nutritional Factors in Psychological Test Behavior," *The Journal of Genetic Psychology* 96 (1960): 343–52.

2.   R. F. Harrell et al., "Can Nutritional Supplements Help Mentally Retarded Children? An Exploratory Study," *Proceedings of the National Academy of Sciences USA* 78, no. 1 (1981): 574–78.

3.   D. Benton and G. Roberts, "Effect of Vitamin and Mineral Supplementation on Intelligence of School Children," *Lancet* 1, no. 8578 (1988): 140–43.

4.   S. J. Schoenthaler et al., "Controlled Trial of Vitamin-Mineral Supplementation: Effects on Intelligence and Performance," *Personality & Individual Differences* 12, no. 4 (1991): 351–52.

5.   D. Benton, "Micro-Nutrient Supplementation and the Intelligence of Children," *Neuroscience and Biobehavioral Reviews* 25, no. 4 (2001): 297–309.

6.   M. Nelson et al., "Nutrient Intakes, Vitamin-Mineral Supplementation and Intelligence in British Schoolchildren," *British Journal of Nutrition* 64, no. 1 (1990): 13–22.

7.   L. J. Whalley et al., "Cognitive Aging, Childhood Intelligence, and the Use of Food Supplements: Possible Involvement of N-3 Fatty Acids," *American Journal of Clinical Nutrition* 80, no. 6 (2004): 1650–57.

8.   W. Snowden, "Evidence from an Analysis of 2000 Errors and Omissions Made in IQ Tests by a Small Sample of Schoolchildren, Undergoing Vitamin and Mineral Supplementation, That Speed of Processing Is an Important Factor in IQ Performance," *Personality & Individual Differences* 22, no. 1 (1997): 131–34.

9. J. Penland, "Zinc Affects Cognition and Psychosocial Function of Middle-School Children" (paper presented at Experimental Biology conference, San Diego, April 4, 2005, pending publication).

10. D. Benton et al., "Thiamine Supplementation, Mood and Cognitive Functioning," *Journal of Pschopharmacology* (Berl) 129, no. 1 (1997): 66–71.

11. P. Willatts et al., "Effect of Long-Chain Polyunsaturated Fatty Acids in Infant Formula on Problem Solving at 10 Months of Age," *Lancet* 352 (1998): 688–91; C. Agostoni et al., "Developmental Quotient at 24 Months and Fatty Acid Composition of Diet in Early Infancy: A Follow Up Study," *Archives of Disease in Childhood* 76, no. 5 (1997): 421–24.

12. AGE 3: C. L. Jensen et al., "Effects of Maternal Docosahexaenoic Acid Intake on Visual Function and Neurodevelopment in Breastfed Term Infants," *American Journal of Clinical Nutrition* 82, no. 1 (2005): 125–32; AGE 4: I. B. Helland et al., "Maternal Supplementation with Very-Long-Chain N-3 Fatty Acids during Pregnancy and Lactation Augments Children's IQ at 4 Years of Age," *Pediatrics* 111, (2003): 39–44.

13. HIGHER IQ: L. Horwood and D. M. Fergusson, "Breastfeeding and Later Cognitive and Academic Outcomes," *Pediatrics* 101 (1998): 1–13; MENTAL HEALTH: C. Lanting et al., "Neurological Differences between 9-Year-Old Children Fed Breast-Milk or Formula-Milk as Babies," *Lancet* 344, no. 13 (1994): 9–22.

Chapter 12

1. D. Benton et al., "Mild Hypoglycaemia and Questionnaire Measures of Aggression," *Biological Psychology* 14, nos. 1–2 (1982): 129–35; M. Colgan and L. Colgan, "Do Nutrient Supplements and Dietary Changes Affect Learning and Emotional Reactions of Children with Learning Difficulties?" *Nutrition and Health* 2, nos. 1–2 (1984): 69–77; J. Goldman et al., "Behavioral Effects of Sucrose on Preschool Children," *Journal of Abnormal Child Psychology* 14, no. 4 (1986): 565–77; M. Lester et al., "Refined Carbohydrate Intake, Hair Cadmium Levels and Cognitive Functioning in Children," *Nutrition and Behavior* 1 (1982): 3–13; S. Schoenthaler et al., "The Impact of a Low Food Additive and Sucrose Diet on Academic Performance in 803 New York City Public Schools," *International Journal of Biosocial and Medical Research* 8, no. 2 (1986): 185–95.

2. C. C. Ani and S. M. Grantham-McGregor, "The Effects of Breakfast on Children's Educational Performance, Attendance and Classroom Behavior," in *Fit for School: How Breakfast Clubs Meet Health, Education and Childcare Needs*, ed.

N. Donovan and C. Street (New Policy Institute, 1999), 14–22; J. L. Brown, "New Findings about Child Nutrition and Cognitive Development," in the same publication, 36–44; C. Michaud et al., "Effects of Breakfast-Size on Short-Term Memory, Concentration, Mood and Blood Glucose," *Journal of Adolescent Health* 12 (1991): 53–57.

3. J. P. Jones, et al., "Choline Availability to the Developing Rat Fetus Alters Adult Hippocampal Long-Term Potentiation," *Developmental Brain Research* 118, nos. 1–2 (1999): 159–67.

4. S. L. Ladd et al., "Effect of Phosphatidylcholine on Explicit Memory," *Clinical Neuropharmacology* 16, no. 6 (1993): 540–49.

5. J. Shabert et al., *The Ultimate Nutrient—Glutamine* (Avery Publications, 1990).

6. T. Ziegler et al., "Safety and Metabolic Effects of L-Glutamine Administration in Humans," *Journal of Parenteral and Enteral Nutrition* 14, no. 4 suppl (1990): 137S–46S.

Chapter 14

1. U.S. Food and Drug Administration, "FDA Proposes New Warnings about Suicidal Thinking, Behavior in Young Adults Who Take Antidepressant Medications," *FDA News* P07-77 (May 2, 2007), www.fda.gov/bbs/topics/NEWS/2007/NEW01624.html.

2. B. Gesch, "Influence of Supplementary Vitamins, Minerals and Essential Fats on the Antisocial Behavior of Young Adult Prisoners," *British Journal of Psychiatry* 181 (2002): 22–28.

3. J. R. Hibbeln, "Fish Consumption and Major Depression," *Lancet* 351 (1998): 1213.

4. B. Nemets et al., "Addition of Omega-3 Fatty Acid to Maintenance Medication Treatment for Recurrent Unipolar Depressive Disorder," *American Journal of Psychiatry* 159 (2002): 477–79; L. Marangell et al., "A Double-Blind, Placebo-Controlled Study of the Omega-3 Fatty Acid Docosahexaenoic Acid (DHA) in the Treatment of Major Depression," *American Journal of Psychiatry* 160, no. 5 (2003): 996–98; A. L. Stoll et al., "Omega 3 Fatty Acids in Bipolar Disorder: A Preliminary Double-Blind, Placebo-Controlled Trial," *Archives of General Psychiatry* 56 (1999): 407–12; M. Maes et al., "Fatty Acid Composition in Major Depression: Decreased w3 Fractions in Cholesteryl Esters and Increased C20:4 Omega 6/C20:5 Omega 3 Ratio in Cholesteryl Esters and Phospholipids," *Journal of Affective Disorders* 38 (1996): 35–46; M. Peet et al., "Depletion of Omega-3

Fatty Acid Levels in Red Blood Cell Membranes of Depressive Patient," *Biological Psychiatry* 43, no. 5 (1998): 315–19.

5. B. Puri et al., "Eicosapentaenoic Acid in Treatment-Resistant Depression," *Archives of General Psychiatry* 59, no. 1 (2002): Letters to the Editor.

6. K. A. Smith et al., "Relapse of Depression after Rapid Depletion of Tryptophan," *Lancet* 349 (1997): 915–19.

7. E. Turner et al., "Serotonin a la carte: Supplementation with the Serotonin Precursor 5-Hydroxytryptophan," *Pharmacology and Therapeutics* 109, no. 3 (2006): 325–38.

8. B. L. Kagan et al., "Oral S-Adenosylmethionine in Depression: A Randomized, Double-Blind, Placebo-Controlled Trial," *American Journal of Psychiatry* 147, no. 5 (1990): 591–95; P. G. Janicak et al., "Parenteral S-adenosyl-methionine (SAMe) in Depression: Literature Review and Preliminary Data," *Psychopharmacology Bulletin* 25, no. 2 (1989): 238–42.

Chapter 15

1. A. Richardson, "Fatty Acids in Dyslexia, Dyspraxia, ADHD and the Autistic Spectrum," *Nutrition Practitioner* 3, no. 3 (2001): 18–24.

2. A. J. Richardson and J. Wilmer, "Association between Fatty Acid Symptoms and Dyslexic and ADHD Characteristics in Normal College Students" (paper given at British Dyslexia Association International Conference, University of York, April 2001); M. H. Jorgensen et al., "Is There a Relation between Docosahexaenoic Acid Concentration in Mothers' Milk and Visual Development in Term Infants?" *Journal of Pediatric Gastroenterology and Nutrition* 32 (2001): 293–96.

3. A. J. Richardson et al., "Fatty Acid Deficiency Signs Predict the Severity of Reading and Related Problems in Dyslexic Children" (paper given at British Dyslexia Association International Conference, University of York, April 2001).

4. C. M. Absolon et al., "Psychological Disturbance in Atopic Eczema: The Extent of the Problem in School-Aged Children," *British Journal of Dermatology* 137, no. 2 (1997): 241–45.

5. A. J. Richardson et al., "Abnormal Cerebral Phospholipid Metabolism in Dyslexia Indicated by Phosphorus-31 Magnetic Resonance Spectroscopy," *NMR in Biomedicine* 10 (1997): 309–14.

6. B. J. Stordy, "Dyslexia, Attention Deficit Hyperactivity Disorder, Dyspraxia—Do Fatty Acids Help?" *Dyslexia Review* 9, no. 2 (1997): 1–3.

7.   B. J. Stordy, "Benefit of Docosahexanoic Acid Supplements to Dark Adaptation in Dyslexics," *Lancet* 346 (1995): 385.

8.   I. D. Capel et al., "Comparison of Concentrations of Some Trace, Bulk, and Toxic Metals in the Hair of Normal and Dyslexic Children," *Clinical Chemistry* 27, no. 6 (1981): 879–81.

Chapter 16

1.   R. J. Prinz et al., "Dietary Correlates of Hyperactive Behavior in Children," *Journal of Consulting and Clinical Psychology* 48 (1980): 760–69; S. J. Schoenthaler et al., "The Effect of Randomised Vitamin-Mineral Supplementation on Violent and Non-violent Antisocial Behaviour among Incarcerated Juveniles," *Journal of Nutritional & Environmental Medicine* 7 (1997): 343–52.

2.   L. Langseth and J. Dowd, "Glucose Tolerance and Hyperkinesis," *Food and Cosmetics Toxicology* 16 (1978): 129.

3.   I. Colquhon and S. Bunday, "A Lack of Essential Fats as a Possible Cause of Hyperactivity in Children," *Medical Hypotheses* 7 (1981): 673–79.

4.   N. Sinn, "Physical Fatty Acid Deficiency Signs in Children with ADHD Symptoms," *Prostaglandins, Leukotrienes, and Essential Fatty Acids* 77, no. 2 (2007): 109–15.

5.   L. J. Stevens et al., "Essential Fat Metabolism in Boys with Attention-Deficit Hyperactivity Disorder," *American Journal of Clinical Nutrition* 65 (1995): 761–68.

6.   J. R. Burgess, "ADHD: Observational and Interventional Studies" (NIH Workshop on Omega-3 EFAs in Psychiatric Disorder, National Institutes of Health, Bethesda, MD, 1998); A. J. Richardson et al., "Treatment with Highly Unsaturated Fatty Acids Can Reduce ADHD Symptoms in Children with Specific Learning Difficulties: A Randomised Controlled Trial" (paper given at British Dyslexia Association International Conference, University of York, April 2001); A. Richardson and B. Puri, "A Randomized Double-Blind, Placebo-Controlled Study of the Effects of Supplementation with Highly Unsaturated Fatty Acids on ADHD-Related Symptoms in Children with Specific Learning Difficulties," *Progress in Neuro-Psychopharmacology & Biological Psychiatry* 26, no. 2 (2002): 233–39.

7.   N. Sinn and J. Bryan, "Effect of Supplementation with Polyunsaturated Fatty Acids and Micronutrients on Learning and Behavior Problems Associated with Child ADHD," *Journal of Developmental & Behavioral Pediatrics* 28, no. 2 (2007): 82–91.

8. A. Richardson and B. Puri, "A Randomized Double-Blind, Placebo-Controlled Study of the Effects of Supplementation with Highly Unsaturated Fatty Acids on ADHD," *Progress in Neuro-Psychopharmacology & Biological Psychiatry* 26, no. 2 (2002): 233–39.

9. B. O'Reilly, Hyperactive Children's Support Group Conference, London, June 2001.

10. M. D. Boris and F. S. Mandel, "Foods and Additives Are Common Causes of the Attention Deficit Hyperactive Disorder in Children," *Annals of Allergy* 72 (1994): 462–68.

11. R. J. Theil, "Nutrition Based Interventions for ADD and ADHD," *Townsend Letter for Doctors & Patients* 201 (April 2000): 93–95.

12. A. R. Swain et al., "Salicylates, Oligoantigenic Diet and Behavior," *Lancet* 2, no. 8445 (1985): 41–42.

13. B. Starobrat-Hermelin and T. Kozielec, "The Effects of Magnesium Physiological Supplementation on Hyperactivity in Children with Attention Deficit Hyperactivity Disorder (ADHD): Positive Response to Magnesium Oral Loading Test," *Magnesium Research* 10, no. 2 (1997): 149–56.

14. N. I. Ward, "Assessment of Clinical Factors in Relation to Child Hyperactivity," *Journal of Nutritional & Environmental Medicine* 7 (1997): 333–42.

15. N. I. Ward, "Hyperactivity and a Previous History of Antibiotic Usage," *Nutrition Practitioner* 3, no. 3 (2001): 12.

16. S. J. Schoenthaler et al., "The Effect of Randomised Vitamin-Mineral Supplementation on Violent and Non-violent Antisocial Behaviour among Incarcerated Juveniles," *Journal of Nutritional & Environmental Medicine* 7 (1997): 343–52.

17. N. D. Volkow et al., "Therapeutic Doses of Oral Methylphenidate Significantly Increase Extracellular Dopamine in the Human Brain," *Journal of Neuroscience* 21, no. RC121 (2001): 1–5.

18. J. Baizer, Annual Meeting of the Society for Neuroscience, 11 November 2001.

19. R. D. Ciaranello, "Attention Deficit-Hyperactivity Disorder and Resistance to Thyroid Hormone—A New Idea?" *New England Journal of Medicine* 328, no. 14 (1993): 1038–39.

20. National Institutes of Health, *NIH Consensus Statement: Diagnosis and Treatment of Attention Deficit Hyperactivity Disorder (ADHD)* (NIH, 1998).

21. N. Lambert and C. Hartsough, "Prospective Study of Tobacco Smoking and Substance Dependencies among Samples of ADHD and Non-ADHD Participants," *Journal of Learning Disabilities* 31 (1998): 533–44.

22. See the Optimal Wellness Center website, www.mercola.com/2001/jan/7/lendon_smith.htm.

23. K. Blum and J. Holder, *The Reward Deficiency Syndrome* (American College of Addictionology and Compulsive Disorders, Amereol Ltd., 2002).

24. N. D. Volkow et al., "Therapeutic Doses of Oral Methylphenidate Significantly Increase Extracellular Dopamine in the Human Brain," *Journal of Neuroscience* 21, no. 2 (2001): 121.

Chapter 17

1. B. Rimland et al., "The Effect of High Doses of Vitamin B6 on Autistic Children: A Double-Blind Crossover Study," *American Journal of Psychiatry* 135, no. 4 (1978): 472–75.

2. S. I. Pfeiffer et al., "Efficacy of Vitamin B6 and Magnesium in the Treatment of Autism: A Methodology Review and Summary of Outcomes," *Journal of Autism and Developmental Disorders* 25, no. 5 (1995): 481–93.

3. J. Martineau et al., "Vitamin B6, Magnesium, and Combined B6-Mg: Therapeutic Effects in Childhood Autism," *Biological Psychiatry* 20, no. 5 (1985): 467–78.

4. S. Vancassel et al., "Plasma Fatty Acid Levels in Autistic Children," *Prostaglandins, Leukotrienes, and Essential Fatty Acids* 65 (2001): 1–7.

5. J. G. Bell et al., "Red Blood Cell Fatty Acid Compositions in a Patient with Autism Spectrum Disorder: A Characteristic Abnormality in Neurodevelopmental Disorders?" *Prostaglandins, Leukotrienes, and Essential Fatty Acids* 63, nos. 1–2 (2000): 21–25; J. G. Bell, "Fatty Acid Deficiency and Phospholipase A2 in Autistic Spectrum Disorders" (workshop report, St Anne's College, Oxford, September 2001).

6. M. Megson, "Is Autism a G-Alpha Protein Defect Reversible with Natural Vitamin A?" *Medical Hypotheses* 54, no. 6 (2000): 979–83.

7. M. Megson, "The Biological Basis for Perceptual Deficits in Autism: Vitamin A and G-Proteins" (lecture given at Ninth International Symposium on Functional Medicine, May 2002).

8. P. Whiteley, "The Biology of Autism—Unravelled" (presentation given at the Autism Unravelled Conference, London, May 2001).

9. P. Whitely et al., "A Gluten-Free Diet as an Intervention for Autism and Associated Spectrum Disorders: Preliminary Findings," *Autism: International Journal of Research and Practice* 3 (1999): 45–65.

10. W. G. Crook, "Anti-Fungal Drugs More Helpful Than Ritalin in Autistic Children," letter to the editor, *Townsend Letter for Doctors & Patients* 213 (April 2001): 99.

11. A. J. Wakefield et al., "Enterocolitis in Children with Developmental Disorders," *American Journal of Gastroenterology* 95, no. 9 (2000): 2285–95.

12. M. A. Brudnak, "Application of Genomeceuticals to the Molecular and Immunological Aspects of Autism," *Medical Hypotheses* 57, no. 2 (2001): 186–91.

13. P. Varmanen et al., "X-Prolyl Dipeptidyl Aminopeptidase Gene (PepX) Is Part of the GlnrA Operon in *Lactobacillus rhamnosus*," *Journal of Bacteriology* 182, no. 1 (2000): 146–54.

14. P. Whitely et al., "A Gluten-Free Diet as an Intervention for Autism and Associated Spectrum Disorders: Preliminary Findings," *Autism: International Journal of Research and Practice* 3 (1999): 45–65.

15. J. R. Cade, University of Florida Department of Medicine and Physiology, at http://paleodiet.com/autism/cadelet.txt.

16. M. Ash and E. Gilmore, "Modifying Autism through Functional Nutrition" (paper given at Allergy Research Group conference, London, January 2001).

17. Graph based, with permission, on data from Table 4 of the following article: J. R. Cade, R. M. Privette, et al., "Autism and Schizophrenia: Intestinal Disorders," *Nutritional Neuroscience* 3 (1999): 57–72.

18. R. Waring, "Sulphate, Sulphation and Gut Permeability: Are Cytokines Involved?" (paper presented at Autism Unravelled Conference Proceedings, London, May 11, 2001).

19. A. J. Wakefield et al., "Ileal-Lymphoid Hyperplasia, Non-specific Colitis, and Pervasive Developmental Disorder in Children," *Lancet* 351 (1998): 637–41.

20. A. Wakefield, Allergy Research Foundation conference, November 1999.

21. F. E. Yazbak, "Autism—Is There a Vaccine Connection?" see www.autisme.net/Yazbak1.htm.

22. B. Rimland, "The Autism Epidemic, Vaccinations and Mercury," *Journal of Nutritional & Environmental Medicine* 10 (2000): 261–66.

23. Ibid.; see also Ashcraft & Gerel (law firm), "Autism Caused by Childhood Vaccinations Containing Thimerosal or Mercury," at www.ashcraftandgerel.com/thimerosal.html.

24. B. Rimland, "Parents' Ratings of the Effectiveness of Drugs and Nutrients," *Autism Research Review International* 8 (October 1994).

25. D. B. Smith and E. Obbens, "Antifolate-Antiepileptic Relationships," in *Folic Acid in Neurology, Psychiatry and Internal Medicine*, ed. M. I. Botez and E. H. Reynolds (Raven Press, 1979), 267–83.

26. F. B. Gibberd et al., "The Influence of Folic Acid on the Frequency of Epileptic Attacks," *European Journal of Clinical Pharmacology* 19, no. 1 (1981): 57–60.

27. D. B. Smith and E. Obbens, "Antifolate-Antiepileptic Relationships," in *Folic Acid in Neurology, Psychiatry and Internal Medicine*, ed. M. I. Botez and E. H. Reynolds (Raven Press, 1979), 267–83.

28. M. Nakazawa, "High Dose Vitamin B6 Therapy in Infantile Spasms—The Effect of Adverse Reactions," *Brain and Development* 5, no. 2 (1983): 193.

28. J. Pietz et al., "Treatment of Infantile Spasms with High-Dosage Vitamin B6," *Epilepsia* 34, no. 4 (1993): 757–63.

30. A. Sohler and C. Pfeiffer, "A Direct Method for the Determination of Managanese in Whole Blood: Patients with Seizure Activity Have Low Blood Levels," *Journal of Orthomolecular Psychiatry* 12 (1983): 215–34; C. L. Dupont and Y. Tanka, "Blood Manganese Levels in Children with Convulsive Disorder," *Biochemical Medicine* 33, no. 2 (1985): 246–55; P. S. Papavasiliou et al., "Seizure Disorders and Trace Metals: Manganese Tissue Levels in Treated Epileptics," *Neurology* 29 (1979): 1466.

31. Y. Tanaka, "Low Manganese Level May Trigger Epilepsy," *Journal of the American Medical Association* 238 (1977): 1805.

32. C. Pfeiffer et al., "Zinc and Manganese in the Schizophrenias," *Journal of Orthomolecular Psychiatry* 12 (1983): 215–34.

33. S. K. Gupta et al., "Serum Magnesium Levels in Idiopathic Epilepsy," *Journal of the Association of Physicians of India* 42, no. 6 (1994): 456–57.

34. L. F. Gorges et al., "Effect of Magnesium on Epileptic Foci," *Epilepsia* 19, no. 1 (1978): 81–91.

35. Balla et al., "The Role of Magnesium Deficiency in Convulsive Syndromes in Children," *Pediatria Romania* 31, no. 4 (1982): 343–47.

36. C. L. Zhang et al., "Paroxysmal Epileptiform Discharges in Temporal Lobe Slices after Prolonged Exposure to Low Magnesium Are Resistant to Clinically Used Anticonvulsants," *Epilepsy Research* 20, no. 2 (1995): 105–11.

37. VITAMIN B1: M. I. Botez et al., "Thiamine and Folate Treatment of Chronic Epileptic Patients: A Controlled Study with the Wechsler IQ Scale," *Epilepsy Research* 16, no. 2 (1993): 157–63; A. Keyser, "Epileptic Manifestations and Vitamin B1 Deficiency," *European Neurology* 31, no. 3 (1991): 121–25; SELENIUM: V. T. Ramaeckers, "Selenium Deficiency Triggering Intractable Seizures," *Neuropediatrics* 25, no. 4 (1994): 217–23; VITAMIN E: I. R. Tupeev et al., "The Antioxidant System in the Dynamic Combined Treatment of Epilepsy Patients with Traditional Anticonvulsant Preparations and an Antioxidant—Alpha-Tocopherol," *Biulleten' eksperimental'noĭ biologii i meditsiny* 116, no. 10 (1993): 362–64.

38. F. E. Ali et al., "Loss of Seizure Control Due to Anticonvulsant-Induced Hypocalcemia," *Annals of Pharmacotherapy* 38, no. 6 (2004): 1002–5.

39. Ibid.

40. S. Yehuda, "Essential Fat Preparation (SR-3) Raises the Seizure Threshold in Rats," *European Journal of Pharmacology* 254, nos. 1–2 (1994): 193–98.

41. S. Schlanger et al., "Diet Enriched with Omega-3 Fatty Acids Alleviates Convulsion Symptoms in Epilepsy Patients," *Epilepsia* 43, no. 1 (2002): 103–4.

42. B. K. Puri, "The Safety of Evening Primrose Oil in Epilepsy," *Prostaglandins, Leukotrienes, and Essential Fatty Acids* 77, no. 2 (2007): 101–3.

43. E. S. Roach et al., "N,N-Dimethylglycine for Epilepsy," letter to the editor, *New England Journal of Medicine* 307 (1982): 1081–82.

44. R. Huxtable and H. Laird, "The Prolonged Anticonvulsant Action of Taurine on Genetically Determined Seizure-Susceptibility," *Canadian Journal of Neurological Sciences* 5 (1978): 220.

45. D. A. Richards et al., "Extracellular GABA in the Ventrolateral Thalamus of Rats Exhibiting Spontaneous Absence Epilepsy: A Microdialysis Study," *Journal of Neurochemistry* 65, no. 4 (1995): 1674–80.

46. J. Schmidt, "Comparative Studies on the Anti-Convulsant Effectiveness of Nootropic Drugs in Kindled Rats," *Biomedica Biochimica Acta* 49, no. 5 (1990): 413–19.

Chapter 18

1. B. Gesch, "Influence of Supplementary Vitamins, Minerals and Essential Fats on the Antisocial Behavior of Young Adult Prisoners," *British Journal of Psychiatry* 181 (2002): 22–28.

2. T. Hamazaki et al., "The Effect of Docosahexaenoic Acid on Aggression in Young Adults: A Placebo-Controlled Double-Blind Study," *Journal of Clinical Investigation* 97 (1996): 1129–33.

3. S. J. Schoenthaler et al., "The Effect of Randomised Vitamin-Mineral Supplementation on Violent and Non-violent Antisocial Behaviour among Incarcerated Juveniles," *Journal of Nutritional & Environmental Medicine* 7 (1997): 343–52.

4. HYPERACTIVE CHILDREN: J. Egger et al., "Controlled Trial of Oligoantigenic Treatment in the Hyperkinetic Syndrome," *Lancet* 1, no. 8428 (1985): 540–45; JUVENILE OFFENDERS: A. G. Schauss and C. E. Simonsen, "A Critical Analysis of the Diets of Chronic Juvenile Offenders, Part 1," *Journal of Orthomolecular Psychiatry* 8, no. 3 (1979): 149–57.

5. D. Papalos and J. Papalos, *The Bipolar Child* (Broadway Books, 2000).

Chapter 19

1. K. Hambidge and A. Silverman, "Pica with Rapid Improvement after Dietary Zinc Supplementation," *Archives of Disease in Childhood* 48 (1973): 567.

2. R. Bakan, "The Role of Zinc in Anorexia Nervosa: Etiology and Treatment," *Medical Hypotheses* 5, no. 7 (1979): 731–36.

3. D. Horrobin and S. C. Cunnane, "Interactions between Zinc, Essential Fatty Acids and Prostaglandins: Relevance to Acrodermatitis Enteropatica, Total Parenteral Nutrition, and Glucagonoma Syndrome, Diabetes, Anorexia Nervosa, and Sickle Cell Anemia," *Medical Hypothesis* 6 (1980): 277–96.

4. R. C. Casper et al., "An Evaluation of Trace Metals, Vitamins and Minerals and Taste Function in Anorexia Nervosa," *American Journal of Clinical Nutrition* 33 (1980): 1801–8; later confirmed by L. Humphries et al., "Zinc Deficiency and Eating Disorders," *Journal of Clinical Psychiatry* 50, no. 12 (1980): 456–59.

5. P. R. Flanagan, "A Model to Produce Pure Zinc Deficiency in Rats and Its Use to Demonstrate That Dietary Phytate Increases the Excretion of Endogenous Zinc," *Journal of Nutrition* 114 (1984): 493–502; A. Grider et al., "Age-Dependent Influence of Dietary Zinc Restriction on Short-Term Memory in Male Rats," *Physiology and Behavior* 72, no. 3 (2001): 339–48.

6. A. Arcasoy et al., "Ultrastructural Changes in the Mucosa of the Small Intestine in Patients with Geophagia (Prasad's Syndrome)," *Journal of Pediatric Gastroenterology and Nutrition* 11, no. 2 (1990): 279–82.

7. D. Bryce-Smith and R. I. Simpson, "Case of Anorexia Nervosa Responding to Zinc Sulphate," *Lancet* 2, no. 8398 (1984): 350.

8. R. L. Katz et al., "Zinc Deficiency in Anorexia Nervosa," *Journal of Adolescent Health Care* 8 (1987): 400–406.

9. L. Humphries et al., "Zinc Deficiency and Eating Disorders," *Journal of Clinical Psychiatry* 50, no. 12 (1989): 456–59.

10. N. F. Shay and H. F. Mangian, "Neurobiology of Zinc-Influenced Eating Behavior," *Journal of Nutrition* 130, no. 5S suppl (2000): 1493S–99S.

11. R. Bakan et al., "Dietary Zinc Intake of Vegetarian and Non-vegetarian Patients with Anorexia Nervosa," *International Journal of Eating Disorders* 13, no. 2 (1993): 229–33.

12. F. Askenazy et al., "Whole Blood Serotonin Content, Tryptophan Concentrations, and Impulsivity in Anorexia Nervosa," *Biological Psychiatry* 43, no. 3 (1998): 188–95.

13. A. Favaro, "Tryptophan Levels, Excessive Exercise, and Nutritional Status in Anorexia Nervosa," *Psychosomatic Medicine* 62, no. 4 (2000): 535–38.

14. P. J. Cowen and K. A. Smith, "Serotonin, Dieting, and Bulimia Nervosa," *Advances in Experimental Medicine and Biology* 467 (1999): 101–4.

Chapter 20

1. Y. Harrison and J. A. Horne, "Sleep Deprivation Affects Speech," *Sleep* 20, no. 10 (1997): 871–77.

2. L. Ozturk et al., "Effects of 48 Hours Sleep Deprivation on Human Immune Profile," *Sleep Research Online* 2, no. 4 (1999): 107–11.

3. J. Owens et al., "Television-Viewing Habits and Sleep Disturbance in School Children," *Pediatrics* 104, no. 3 (1999): 27.

4. L. Hillert et al., "The Effects of 884 MHz GSM Wireless Communication Signals on Headache and Other Symptoms: An Experimental Provocation Study," *Bioelectromagnetics* 29, no. 3: 185–96.

5. M. G. Smits et al., "Melatonin for Chronic Sleep Onset Insomnia in Children: A Randomized Placebo-Controlled Trial," *Journal of Child Neurology* 16, no. 2 (2001): 86–92; E. J. Pavonen et al., "Effectiveness of Melatonin in the Treatment of Sleep Disturbances in Children with Asperger Disorder," *Journal of Child and Adolescent Psychopharmacology* 13, no. 1 (2003): 83–95.

Chapter 21

1. American Dietetic Association, "Promotion of Breastfeeding," *Journal of the American Dietetic Association* 97 (1997): 662–66.

2. J. W. Anderson et al., "Breast-feeding and Cognitive Development: A Meta-analysis," *American Journal of Clinical Nutrition* 70, no. 4 (1999): 525–35.

3. E. L. Mortensen et al., "The Association between Duration of Breastfeeding and Adult Intelligence," *Journal of the American Medical Association* 287 (2002): 2365–71.

4. F. Martinez, "Evaluation of Plasma Tocopherols in Relation to Hematological Indices of Brazilian Infants on Human Milk and Cows' Milk Regime from Birth to 1 Year of Age," *American Journal of Clinical Nutrition* 41, no. 3 (1985): 969.

5. W. Craig, "Plasma Manganese Levels of Human Milk-Fed and Formula-Fed Infants," *Nutrition Reports International* 30, no. 4 (1984): 1003.

6. J. Armstrong et al., "Breastfeeding and Lowering the Risk of Childhood Obesity," *Lancet* 359, no. 9322 (2002): 2003–4.

7. N. I. Ward, "Hyperactivity and a Previous History of Antibiotic Usage," *Nutrition Practitioner* 3, no. 3 (2001): 12.

8. N. I. Ward, "Assessment of Clinical Factors in Relation to Child Hyperactivity," *Journal of Nutritional & Environmental Medicine* 7 (1997): 333–42.

9. R. L. William et al., "Use of Antibiotics in Preventing Recurrent Acute Otitis Media and in Treating Otitis Media with Effusion," *Journal of the American Medical Association* 270 (1993): 1344–51.

10. J. Braly and R. Hoggan, *Dangerous Grains* (Avery, 2002), 24.

Index

A

AA (arachidonic acid), 42

Abbreviations, viii

Absolon, Christine, 129

Acetylcholine, 48, 53, 63, 105–6

Adderall, 139

ADHD (attention deficit/hyperactivity disorder)

allergies and, 80, 81, 136–37

bipolar disorder and, 165–66

causative factors for, 131

checklist for, 132–33

consequences of, 131

deficiencies and, 137–39

dyslexia/dyspraxia and, 126, 127

essential fats and, 36, 134–36

heavy metals and, 139

prevalence of, 131

recommendations for, 142

reward deficiency syndrome and, 141–42

Ritalin for, 139–41

sugar and, 18, 133–34

Adrenaline, 12, 52, 53–121, 119, 122

Agave nectar, 27

Aggression, 80, 162–66

Allergies

ADHD and, 136–37

autism and, 147–52

common foods for, 83–84

definition of, 81–82

digestive problems and, 85

food intolerances and sensitivities vs., 81–83

IgE vs. IgG, 82, 83

prevalence of, 80

preventing, 183–86

symptoms of, 80–81

testing for, 84–86

Allura red AC, 75

Almonds, 56

Alpha-linolenic acid, 40, 41

Aluminum, 69, 70

Amino acids. *See also individual amino acids*

deficiency of, 51

epilepsy and, 159

essential, 54

guidelines for, 57

importance of, 51

neurotransmitters and, 12–13, 52–53, 123–24

supplementing with, 57

Anger, 117

Anorexia, 167–74

Anthocyanidins, 65

Antibiotics, 148, 185–86

Antidepressants, 53, 116

Antinutrients, 13, 73

Antioxidants, 63–65

Aspartame, 26, 75

Asperger's syndrome, 143

Asthma, 75–77

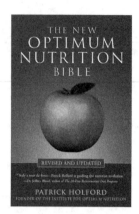